The Remarkable Story of Vaccines

This remarkable book tells you everything you need to know about vaccines. Having nearly forty years' experience of the subject, the author covers the history of vaccines, how they work, how research is carried out, their safety, how they are used in society, the inside track on COVID-19 and what the future holds. It is a deeply personal account, with anecdotes involving a cow called Blossom, a hospital in the Caribbean, a crocodile-infested lake in Malawi, an encounter with Russian soldiers in Prague and many others. An A-to-Z section covers every vaccine from Anthrax to Yellow Fever. It will educate, entertain and enlighten the vaccine scientific community and public health practitioners.

Key Features

- Explores a highly topical concept of vaccines in a comprehensive and easy-to-read manner
- Engages readers with relatable and interesting anecdotes
- Provides a balanced, factual counter to the huge amount of current vaccine misinformation

The Remarkable Story of Vaccines
Vaccines
Milkmaid to Genome

Norman Begg

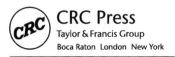

CRC Press
Taylor & Francis Group
Boca Raton London New York

CRC Press is an imprint of the
Taylor & Francis Group, an **informa** business

First edition published 2023
by CRC Press
6000 Broken Sound Parkway NW, Suite 300, Boca Raton, FL 33487-2742

and by CRC Press
4 Park Square, Milton Park, Abingdon, Oxon, OX14 4RN

CRC Press is an imprint of Taylor & Francis Group, LLC

Library of Congress Cataloging-in-Publication Data
Names: Begg, Norman T., author.
Title: The remarkable story of vaccines : milkmaid to genome / by Dr Norman
Begg MBChB DTM & H FFPH.
Description: First edition. | Boca Raton, FL : CRC Press, 2023. | Includes
index. | Summary: "This remarkable book tells you everything you need to
know about vaccines. Having nearly 40 years' experience of the subject,
the author covers the history of vaccines, how they work, how research
is carried out, their safety, how they are used in society, the inside
track on COVID-19, and what the future holds"-- Provided by publisher.
Identifiers: LCCN 2022018398 (print) | LCCN 2022018399 (ebook) | ISBN
9781032301983 (hardback) | ISBN 9781032301976 (paperback) | ISBN
9781003303879 (ebook)
Subjects: LCSH: Vaccines--History. | Vaccination--History.
Classification: LCC QR189 .B44 2023 (print) | LCC QR189 (ebook) | DDC
615.3/72--dc23/eng/20220428
LC record available at https://lccn.loc.gov/2022018398
LC ebook record available at https://lccn.loc.gov/2022018399

ISBN: 978-1-032-30198-3 (hbk)
ISBN: 978-1-032-30197-6 (pbk)
ISBN: 978-1-003-30387-9 (ebk)

DOI: 10.1201/9781003303879

Typeset in Minion Pro
by SPi Technologies India Pvt Ltd (Straive)

In the world of today, true science is much more exciting than fiction can hope to be.

Sir Patrick Moore

Contents

Acknowledgements

This book wouldn't have been possible without the help of many people. Firstly, my friends and family who inspired me to write it in the first place and provided support along the way. My children Sara, Victoria and Lily, reviewed chapters, shared personal experiences and kept me down to earth. My wife Jenny read the book several times and provided a great deal of useful advice (particularly stopping me from me writing medical gobbledegook).

Michael Nelmes gave me precious insights into the life of his great, great, great, great grandmother, Sarah, who provided Edward Jenner with the material for his smallpox vaccine experiment. Kazia Vaughan and Owen Gower of the Edward Jenner Museum helped me fill out the story of that historic event. Cecile Barnich and Robyn Widenmaier of GlaxoSmithKline Vaccines supplied many facts and figures about vaccine trials and Mauro Bernuzzi, former supply chain head at GlaxoSmithKline Vaccines, provided invaluable information about manufacturing and assisted me with the title of the book. Nigel Cunliffe from the Liverpool School of Tropical Medicine and Desiree Witte from the Vaccine Clinical Trial unit in Blantyre, Malawi, sent me the wonderful materials that were used to publicise the rotavirus vaccine trial there, along with personal anecdotes. Stephen Church from Becton Dickinson sent me background information and scientific publications on vaccine needles.

Four of the chapter titles were inspired by personal quotes; for these I would like to thank John McGrath, former head of manufacturing at GlaxoSmithKline Vaccines ("The Space Shuttle"), Euan Ross, professor emeritus of paediatrics at the Royal Free Hospital in London ("It's Not the Vicar's Fault!"), Jeff Almond, former head of research at Sanofi Pasteur ("I'd Rather Be Jabbed Than Shot") and Eric Tayag, former health secretary of the Philippines ("Vaccines Don't Save Lives, Vaccination Does").

I have worked with hundreds of incredible colleagues over the years. I would like to thank all of them; my collective experiences with them provided the material for this book. There are also countless more people who took part in my research over the years, to whom I owe a debt of gratitude that cannot be measured. Finally, the boy with diphtheria, who started me on my journey into the remarkable world of vaccines.

Norman Begg

Author

Norman Begg, MBChB, DTM&H, FFPH, is a public health physician with nearly forty years clinical and research experience in the prevention and control of infectious disease. He has led the development and introduction of several new vaccines in the private and the public sectors.

From 1980 to 1981, he worked as a community paediatrician, running vaccine clinics in a deprived area of London. He worked for fifteen years at the Communicable Disease Surveillance Centre, the UK National Public Health Institute, where he was responsible for surveillance of all vaccine-preventable diseases and conducted trials leading to the successful introduction of several vaccines, particularly those for meningitis. He was head of the Immunisation Division, and also served as deputy director of the Centre for three years. He was a regular consultant to the World Health Organization, and chairman of their European Immunisation Advisory Group. He also worked at the US Centers for Disease Control and Prevention during this time.

At GlaxoSmithKline Vaccines from 2000 to 2017, he held several leadership roles, including head of clinical development for paediatric vaccines, head of scientific affairs and public health, and chief medical officer. He worked on many vaccines, including rotavirus, meningococcal disease, pneumococcal disease and pandemic influenza. He chaired the company's safety board.

Since 2018, he has worked as an independent consultant, providing scientific advice on vaccine research and development, including COVID-19, to pharmaceutical companies and investors.

He has published extensively on the epidemiology, prevention and control of vaccine-preventable disease. He co-edited the *Green Book*, the handbook that describes UK vaccine policy from 1992 to 1996.

A Boy with Diphtheria

"Doc! We got a boy with asthma. He's real sick, better come quick." I arrived in the casualty department minutes later. I was perspiring from the sweltering tropical heat that my body would take several more months to tolerate. Outside, rain battered down relentlessly on the corrugated iron hospital roof, bouncing off the pavement, creating instant puddles and muddy-brown rivers. People huddled together under the hospital eaves, except two young Rastafarians, who splashed about like gleeful schoolboys. I was in Victoria Hospital on the Caribbean island of St Lucia. It was September 1977, rainy season, and I had arrived a few days earlier as a young doctor, fresh from completing my medical training in Edinburgh.

Victoria Hospital was the island's social hub, and the casualty department was where the action was at. Patients would walk for hours from remote villages and sit patiently on wooden benches to be seen by the duty doctor. The hospital sat on top of a hill, with spectacular views of lush, mountainous rainforest. The winding pot-holed approach road up the hill passed through a jumble of bougainvillea, hibiscus, bird of paradise, mango trees, majestic palms, endless banana plants and their starchier cousins, plantains. At the hospital entrance, women with bright headscarves and personalities to match, sold fiery chicken rotis and Accra, a salty fish cake. Patients would arrive with their families, friends and well-wishers. Crowds of onlookers would come to see what the doctor on duty was up to. I got used to several pairs of eyes peeking round the curtain while I stitched up someone who had sliced open their hand while wielding a cutlass – the universal garden tool. This was a far cry from the Royal Infirmary of Edinburgh.

The patient with "asthma" was a boy, about eighteen months old, who was clearly having dif-ficulty breathing. One of my medical house jobs had been working in a unit that specialised in treating asthma, so I was feeling pretty confident as I arrived to see him. My confidence started to evaporate as I examined the boy. Sure enough, he had the breathing distress that is typical of someone with a severe asthma attack, and I could hear what sounded like the characteristic wheezing noise when he breathed out. But as I started to examine him, I realised that this was not a typical case of asthma. The wheezing sound wasn't coming from his chest, but from his throat, as if there was something obstructing the outflow of air. When I listened to his chest through my stethoscope, I didn't hear the whistling noises (doctors call them "rhonchi") that you usually hear in someone with asthma. I could see that his throat was swollen, and there was something at the back which was causing the obstruction. It didn't have the angry red appear-ance of a throat infection. He had a fever, which isn't typical of asthma. I was stumped. I decided to call Dr Ed.

Dr Ed – Ed Cooper – was a British paediatrician who had lived and worked in St Lucia for several years. He had transformed the care of children there. Ed set up vaccination services, development checks and health education for young mothers. Many mothers in St Lucia were no more than children themselves, and the father was often absent. Thanks to Ed Cooper, every child on the island had a child health passport, where all their important health information was stored. When a child was brought to hospital or one of the health centres on the island, the first

DOI: 10.1201/9781003303879-1

question was always: "Did you bring the child's health passport?" A hospital administrator once described Ed to me as someone who can treat you without medicine. That summed him up perfectly. Ed was the first doctor I met who understood that improving health is not just about treating patients. He went on to become a leading authority in Caribbean child health.

"Diphtheria," Ed pronounced the word slowly and emphatically. He had made the diagnosis as soon as he saw the child. The noise that I thought sounded like wheezing was in fact something called stridor. This is the noise that a person makes when their breathing is obstructed in the upper part of their airways. It is a typical sign of diphtheria. The obstruction that I had seen at the back of the boy's throat was a grey - coloured membrane, also typical of diphtheria. So was the fever.

I was dumbfounded. Diphtheria was a disease I had read about in my medical training. It used to be a common cause of death in young children. In 1914, at the outbreak of World War I, 59,324 cases of and 5,863 deaths from diphtheria were recorded in England and Wales. Within ten years, a vaccination against diphtheria had been developed and started to be widely used with dramatic impact. By 1952, the year I was born, the disease had been all but eliminated. Most doctors in developed countries will never see a case nowadays. Diphtheria had been conquered; but not quite.

Back in casualty, things were not going well.

"He needs antitoxin," muttered Ed. The boy had advanced diphtheria. His symptoms were being caused by the powerful toxin that is released by the bacterium that causes diphtheria. Diphtheria toxin is extraordinarily potent. It destroys heart and liver tissue and paralyses the nervous system. Seven - millionths of a gram is enough to kill an adult. The only way to reverse this is by giving a specific diphtheria antitoxin, which can neutralise its effects. Ed asked me to call the pharmacist.

The pharmacy of Victoria Hospital bore no resemblance to the gleaming well-stocked facility I was used to in Edinburgh. There were a mere handful of drugs available. If you needed to give someone a blood transfusion you would be lucky to find any blood there at all. Most blood donations came from the relatives that brought patients to hospital, with a hasty cross match to check compatibility. If I needed a lot of blood, I would go on the radio and ask for volunteers to come to casualty. Amazingly, the pharmacy did have one vial of diphtheria antitoxin. Ed looked at it suspiciously. It didn't have a dose, or an expiry date written on it. He reckoned it was probably a very small dose which was hopelessly out of date. But there was no choice. If we were going to reverse the effects of the toxin that was starting to take over the boy's heart and nervous system, it was our only option. He injected the contents into a vein. Over the next few hours, we gave the best supportive care we could manage, but his symptoms got worse, and he died a few hours later. To this day I remember the feeling of helplessness at not being able to save his life. The feeling of ignorance at not recognising the disease. And the feeling of injustice that he need not have died at all. His child health passport confirmed that he had not been vaccinated. This was the "Aha!" moment. I felt something I had not felt in all the years of lectures, tutorials, rote learning and ward rounds of my medical training: scientific curiosity. I wanted to understand more. I had questions about vaccination, infectious diseases and what could be done to prevent deaths like the one I just witnessed.

I spent more than two years on St Lucia. It was amazing. I saw more illnesses that I had only read about in textbooks: dengue fever, malnutrition, every kind of imaginable worm infestation. I came to realise that there is much more to medicine than prescribing drugs. During my time there, a deadly tropical parasitic disease – bilharzia, also called schistosomiasis – was eradicated from the island. The effort to rid the island of the disease was led by a research institute funded by the Rockefeller Foundation. I had seen a few cases of bilharzia when I first arrived. I remember one young girl staggering into casualty, pale as a sheet with her abdomen distended like an oversized football. She had lost so much blood that her haemoglobin level was a fifth of the normal level. Treatment with a drug called praziquantel had a part to play in the disease eradication effort, but the biggest factor was something much simpler. In St Lucia, women would wash the family clothes in the gushing rivers that cascaded down from the volcanic peaks that dotted the island. Their children would be with them, playing in the water. What they didn't realise is that the rivers were infested by a snail that carries the bilharzia parasite, which would burrow its way through the children's skin into the blood stream, reaching the liver, lungs, bowel and bladder, wreaking havoc on its journey. The solution was simple – provide communal washing facilities in the villages, so the women and children didn't need to go to the snail-infested rivers. Elimination of a disease by basic hygiene. I also saw first-hand the impact of vaccination on children's health there, thanks to Ed Cooper. Measles and whooping cough were very common when I arrived; they were rare by the time I left. I never saw another case of diphtheria. I started to understand that there is a much bigger picture; a complex relationship between health, behaviour, society and poverty, that went way beyond my conventional medical training. I had discovered the power of prevention. The great polymath Benjamin Franklin once said "An ounce of prevention is worth a pound of cure." I don't think I would have seen this bigger picture so clearly if I had stayed in Edinburgh and followed a classical, safe medical career path. When I told one of the consultants at Edinburgh Royal Infirmary that I was going to work in the Caribbean, he thought I was crazy. "You'll never get a job when you come back!" he boomed. "You'll be out of the system." (Whatever that meant). He was wrong – I had some of the most rewarding jobs in my life after I came back to the UK, but more importantly, I returned from St Lucia a very different sort of doctor, with a more holistic perspective on medicine, and an insatiable curiosity for what makes us ill, and better. Medicine would never be the same for me again.

Over the next forty years, I did many different medical jobs – community paediatrician, general practitioner, infectious disease epidemiologist, researcher. Vaccination was always a common thread – from giving vaccines to babies in South East London, to investigating outbreaks of measles and meningitis, to research on new vaccines – rotavirus, pandemic flu, malaria and others. It all started from the boy with diphtheria.

2

The Milkmaid's Legacy

Sarah Nelmes looked at her right hand with a mixture of resignation and anticipation. The large, raised blister next to her thumb was a familiar sight. It was cowpox. It had started a few days earlier as a flat round red sore, which slowly rose up, like a Yorkshire pudding, then blistered. It was 1796, and Sarah was a milkmaid in Berkeley, Gloucestershire. The daughter of Richard Baker, a local farmer, she lived in a small but pristine cottage. Sarah had her father's hazel eyes and wavy black hair, but whereas his skin was wind-whipped, like used sandpaper, Sarah's was perfect alabaster. She had caught cowpox from Blossom, a docile cow that she milked daily. Cowpox was a common occupational hazard for English milkmaids in the eighteenth century. It was transmitted from sores on infected udders, passing to the milkmaids as they squeezed the cow's teats between the thumb and forefinger. It was a mild disease – the blisters would heal in a few days with no permanent effects apart from some scarring. Sarah had managed to escape cowpox, so seeing the blister felt like a rite of passage. But it also meant something much more significant. She was about to take part in an experiment that would change the course of medical history, and lead to the eradication of a deadly disease, smallpox. She called on a local family doctor and surgeon, Edward Jenner. Jenner was the son of a preacher who had started his apprenticeship aged thirteen, under a local surgeon, completing his studies at St George's Hospital in London. Jenner loved nature, played the violin, but above all, had a fierce scientific curiosity. The prestigious Royal Society, the learned society that has existed since 1660 to promote scientific excellence, made him a fellow for his painstaking research on the life of the nesting cuckoo. He described how the newly hatched cuckoo pushed its host's eggs and fledgling chicks out of the nest, contrary to existing belief that the adult cuckoo was the culprit. He published research which advanced the understanding of angina pectoris, the chest pain due to the lack of blood flow to heart muscle. He formed the Gloucester Medical Society, where like-minded doctors exchanged information and debated scientific theories. When Sarah arrived at his home in Berkeley, he was ecstatic. By now, she had two more blisters, on her wrist and index finger. The experiment could begin.

At the time Sarah went to visit Jenner, smallpox was rampant. The disease ravaged eighteenth-century Europe. Four hundred thousand people died from smallpox every year, more than the number that were killed in wars. During epidemics, up to three in ten people who caught the disease would die from it. In young children, four in five succumbed. Those that survived were often left with terrible disfiguring scars. It was called the speckled monster. There was no cure and no way of avoiding it. People tried to protect themselves by deliberately infecting themselves with smallpox – a process called inoculation or variolation. Pus from a person with smallpox was inserted under the skin, using a small scalpel. This rather draconian practice had originated in China several centuries earlier, where they blew powder from smallpox scabs up the nose. Variolation was introduced to the Western world by a British aristocrat who rejoiced in the name of Lady Mary Wortley Montagu. She and her brother had both contracted smallpox. Her brother died of the illness, and while she survived the attack, she was left with

DOI: 10.1201/9781003303879-2

terrible scarring. She learned about variolation in Constantinople (now Istanbul), where her husband had been ambassador to the Ottoman Empire. She had both her children variolated – one in Turkey in 1718, and the other in 1721 when she returned to England; the first person in the country to have the procedure. The same year, six prisoners at Newgate Prison awaiting execution were offered the chance to undergo variolation instead of execution: they all survived and were released. A highly unethical trial by today's standards, but luckily with a successful outcome. Lady Montagu persuaded the Princess of Wales, Caroline of Ansbach, to have the procedure. Royal endorsement made it popular, especially among the upper classes, although there were also very vocal opponents who derided it as "oriental, irreligious and a fad of ignorant women".

Variolation did provide some immunity to smallpox, but it didn't stop the spread of the disease, as a variolated person could pass the disease onto others. It was also a highly dangerous procedure, as it could produce full-blown smallpox – two to three percent of people who were variolated died of the disease. No-one was able to escape smallpox – with one exception. Milkmaids seemed to be immune to smallpox. When an epidemic of smallpox arrived, they miraculously survived – either not catching it all, or having a very mild illness. There are numerous references in art and literature to "the beautiful milkmaid", their skin unblemished by smallpox scars. It was believed that they developed their immunity from catching cowpox while milking their herds. Cowpox is similar to smallpox, but much less severe. It seemed that once exposed to cowpox, the maids were immune to its more unpleasant cousin, smallpox. In 1774, Benjamin Jesty, a farmer from Dorset, decided to protect his family during a smallpox epidemic. He took some pus from the udders of one of his cows that had cowpox, and, using one of his wife's stocking needles, injected his wife and two children. None of them caught smallpox. Jesty wanted to protect his family, but unlike Jenner, he had no interest in the science behind what he had done, and his experiment was never published. He suffered a great deal of abuse from the local community, forcing him and his family to flee their home; it was only thirty years later that his contribution would be acknowledged by the quirkily named Original Vaccine Pock Institute, another learned society.

Dr Jenner wanted to go one step further. He wanted to prove beyond doubt that cowpox could protect against smallpox, and publicise his findings to the medical community. Twenty-two years after Jesty had used cowpox to protect his family, Sarah Nelmes gave Jenner the opportunity to prove his theory.

On May 14, 1796, Jenner scraped some of the pus that was oozing out of Sarah's blisters. With a small surgical scalpel, he made two neat cuts in the forearm of James Phipps, the eight-year-old son of his gardener, and gingerly inserted the pus. Over the following weeks, James developed typical symptoms of cowpox, with red ulcers where Jenner had injected the liquid, inflamed joints, pain in the groin and fever. Luckily, he made a full recovery. Six weeks later, Jenner then deliberately infected James with smallpox, by variolation. Normally, variolation produced a typical smallpox blister, and scarring. James did not develop any of these signs. Over the next few months, Jenner tried several times to infect him with smallpox, but each time he did not develop any symptoms. This was not the most ethical experiment, but it had worked. Dr Jenner wrote up his findings in a pamphlet with the rather long-winded title: "An Inquiry into the Causes and Effects of the *Variolae Vaccinae*, a Disease Discovered in Some of the Western Counties of England, Particularly Gloucestershire, and Known by the Name of the Cow Pox". He used the word "vaccination" to describe his technique, from the Latin word *vacca* which means cow – Sarah's (and Blossom's) legacy. He went on to vaccinate many more people, working from a simple hut in his garden, that he called the Temple of Vaccination. After some initial scepticism, Jenner's work quickly caught on, and smallpox vaccination became established medical practice throughout Europe and North America. Disease rates plummeted. In London, almost 20,000 people had died in the decade before Jenner's experiment. During the decade 1811–1820, less than 8,000 Londoners died from smallpox. The disease continued to decline over the next hundred years, and by the 1950s, it was confined to Africa, Asia and South America. In 1967, the World Health Organization began a concerted effort to eradicate smallpox worldwide. Mass vaccination campaigns began. In remote areas, teams of volunteers went from village to village, vaccinating people and looking for possible cases. Smallpox vaccination leaves a tell-tale scar, so it was easy for the volunteers to know who had already been vaccinated. On October 26, 1977, Ali Maow Maalin, a cook from Somalia, became the last person in the world to develop naturally acquired smallpox. The following year, two people in the UK developed smallpox; the source of their infection was a laboratory in Birmingham that was doing smallpox research. These would be the last cases ever, and on 8 May 1980, the World Health Organization declared that smallpox had been eradicated from the face of the earth. No human being has caught smallpox since then. The virus no longer exists in the wild, so people do not need to be vaccinated anymore. Laboratory stocks of the virus have been systematically destroyed; the virus is now kept in just two laboratories in the world. There is a long-running debate about whether these remaining stocks should be destroyed, and a group of experts meets periodically to revisit the question. For now, they have advised to keep the stocks, largely because of concerns that there may be secret stocks held by rogue or terrorist organisations. In the event of a deliberate release, the original virus would be needed to produce a vaccine once more.

The principle of vaccination – giving someone a mild version of a disease to protect against a more serious version – changed the course of medical history. In the nineteenth century, Louis Pasteur, a combative French microbiologist, set out to exploit this principle to produce other vaccines. He believed that it was possible to weaken a virus or bacterium by repeatedly growing it in an animal. He used the word *attenue* French for mitigate, to describe this. Attenuation is the word now used to describe the process by which viruses and bacteria are weakened to make safe vaccines. He also gave us the word pasteurisation, which is heating liquids for consumption such as milk, in order to kill unwanted bacteria (a good Frenchman, Pasteur also used it to improve the quality of wine). Pasteur's first vaccines were for animal infections – chicken cholera, and sheep anthrax. These were successful, but the vaccine that shot him to fame was rabies. He produced the vaccine by giving the virus to rabbits, cutting their brains into strips after they died, drying them in a jar and grinding them up. On July 6, 1885, he injected his vaccine into Joseph Meister, a nine-year-old schoolboy from the Alsace, who had been attacked by a rabid dog. Pasteur gave him twelve injections over the next several days. The experiment was technically illegal, as Pasteur did not have a medical degree. The boy lived, and Pasteur was hailed as a hero. Streets in towns and cities all over the world are named after him, and the Pasteur Institute is a leading French vaccine research foundation, with a worldwide network of institutes. I've been to the Pasteur Institute in Paris, and as I expected, it was staffed by brilliant researchers who have dedicated their life to vaccine discovery. I also went to Iran a few years ago, where there has been a branch of the Pasteur Institute for over a hundred years. I spent a truly enlightening day with their top scientists. Iran has a rich history of medical science, with medical textbooks dating back over a thousand years and the researchers of the Pasteur Institute are leaders in the region.

One of Pasteur's rivals was Robert Koch, a German doctor. He transformed the science of microbiology and defined the rules that identify the cause of an infectious disease. Koch's rules (or "postulates", as they are known) are still used today. Koch also discovered the bacterium that causes tuberculosis. He tried, unsuccessfully, to make a vaccine, but his work had a huge impact on vaccine development. The Robert Koch Institute in Berlin is Germany's leading infectious disease control centre.

The work of Pasteur and Koch ushered in the "golden era" of vaccination. Over the next fifty years, vaccines would be developed for tetanus, diphtheria, typhoid fever, tuberculosis, whooping cough, yellow fever and others. Tetanus and diphtheria antitoxins were also created; they didn't prevent the diseases, but if given quickly could stop you from dying. Scientists began to collaborate internationally and across disciplines: diphtheria antitoxin was discovered by an aristocratic Japanese physician, Kitasato Shibasaburo, and a German physiologist, Emil von Behring (he got a Nobel prize, Kitasato didn't).

War was often the major driving force behind these early discoveries. Soldiers would be vaccinated to keep them fighting fit. Napoleon had already worked this out a century earlier, ordering all his troops to be vaccinated against smallpox. After losing at Waterloo, his troops refused to be vaccinated, in an act of defiance against his dictatorship. This resulted in a resurgence of the disease and contributed to their loss of the Franco–Prussian War. During World War I, thousands of lives were saved by vaccinating allied troops against typhoid. This success would, however, be dwarfed by another infectious disease that would follow after the war was over. The influenza pandemic of 1918–1920 killed between 20 and 50 million people, more than had died during the entire conflict. There was no vaccine and no treatment and although a virus was suspected as being the cause, the technology did not exist to confirm it. The influenza virus was first isolated in 1933, by a team of researchers from the UK Medical Research Council. The staff gathered nasal fluids and throat garglings from a sick researcher, filtered them, and dripped them into ferrets. Within forty-eight hours, the ferrets would start sneezing and displaying signs of an influenza-like disease. It would take many more years to discover that there was more than one strain of the virus. The first vaccine that contained the two main strains, type A and B, began clinical trials in 1942 and started to be used in 1945.

After World War II, the focus of vaccine research turned to civilians. The first disease to be tackled was polio. Polio epidemics were rife in the 1950s, leaving thousands of people paralysed, kept alive by living in an iron lung. Imagine spending your life, lying on a bed, with a metal cage over your chest, without which you couldn't breathe. There is a famous photograph taken in a Los Angeles hospital, with row upon row of polio victims, trapped forever in their iron cages. Although the disease affects the nervous system, it is actually a gut infection; people get infected by coming into contact with the virus, which is excreted in the stools of people who have the disease. The virus can survive in sewage and water; during polio epidemics, parents would ban their children from public swimming pools for fear of them contracting the virus.

In 1954, the first trial of a polio vaccine produced by Jonas Salk began. Jonas Salk, raised in the Bronx, was the son of Jewish immigrants. His outstanding academic ability was spotted early, earning him a place at the City College of New York where he studied chemistry, followed by a medical degree at New York University. There was a lot riding on Salk's trial, in which 1.8 million children received either the vaccine, or a placebo. The trial showed it was 80–90% effective against polio, and it started to be used immediately. A few years later another American, Albert Sabin, developed a version that could be given by mouth (oral). Sabin, also the son of Jewish immigrants, had attended the same medical school as Salk. Despite their similar backgrounds and shared scientific interest, they never saw eye to eye. Salk passionately believed his injected vaccine was superior, as it did not carry the small risk of paralysis that was seen with Sabin's oral vaccine. Sabin was unable to acknowledge this risk (which was real). Nevertheless, both vaccines become widely adopted and within a few years, polio was virtually eliminated in the Western world. In 1988, the World Health Organization again embarked on a mission to eradicate the disease worldwide. At that time, polio still paralysed a thousand children a day in the developing world. The availability of the oral vaccine meant that mass campaigns could be carried out on an unprecedented scale. The scale of these campaigns is mind-boggling. During a typical campaign in India – called National Immunisation Day – more than 2 million volunteers went from house to house, giving two drops of the vaccine directly into the mouth of every child under the age of five. That's 172 million children in one day. Even the best efforts of mass COVID-19 vaccination in countries like Israel and the UK pale into insignificance by comparison. Today, there are less than 500 cases of polio a year worldwide, and the naturally occurring disease exists in only two countries, Afghanistan and Pakistan. These last bastions are hampered by an unstable security situation, and governments that have little control over large swathes of the countries. The global polio eradication effort has the support of many agencies and donors but also front-line volunteers, notably from Rotary International through their PolioPlus programme.

The early days of polio vaccination weren't all plain sailing. One of the first companies licensed to produce Salk's polio vaccine in the United States was Cutter Laboratories. In April 1955, they produced batches of vaccine in which the polio virus had not been properly killed. Children were injected with living, un-modified polio virus. It was one of the worst pharmaceutical disasters in history. Forty thousand suffered mild polio, there were 200 cases of permanent paralysis and ten deaths from the faulty vaccine.

Despite the Cutter setback, vaccine research continued apace. Many childhood illnesses became diseases of the past – measles, mumps, rubella, chickenpox, meningitis and rotavirus, a common cause of childhood diarrhoea. Maurice Hilleman, the eighth child of Montana farmers, developed no fewer than eight of the fourteen vaccines used in today's US childhood vaccination schedule. He was not a medical doctor, having completed a degree in microbiology at the University of Chicago. He was a forceful personality but also modest – none of his vaccines or discoveries are named after him. The only lasting connection to his family is his daughter, Jeryl Lyn. He isolated the mumps virus from her when she had the illness and used it to develop a vaccine. More than fifty years later, the mumps vaccine is still developed with the Jeryl Lyn strain, which is preserved in continuous culture, rather like yoghurt.

Adults also benefited from vaccine discoveries such as influenza, hepatitis and pneumonia. The pneumonia vaccine was the brainchild of Robert Austrian, a brilliant microbiologist. He worked out that the causative organism, *Streptococcus pneumoniae* – the pneumococcus – existed as many different strains. He managed to identify eighty-three – pretty good, as there are only about a hundred altogether. He ran a legendary trial on South African gold miners, which showed the vaccine worked, and pneumococcal vaccine is now a standard recommended vaccine for older adults. I met Professor Austrian – "Bob" as he insisted everyone call him – at a World Health Organization meeting in Geneva. I had been asked to write the notes of the meeting – the "rapporteur" – and was pretty nervous in the presence of such a giant. He was one of the most unassuming, courteous people I had ever met, but the bit that endeared me to him most was when he described the pneumococcus as a bacterium with "charm".

More recently, vaccines have been developed for human papillomavirus (the cause of cervical cancer), dengue fever, malaria, shingles, Ebola and of course, COVID-19. There are now vaccines for thirty-three diseases (see A-to-Z of Vaccines). I've had fourteen of them, including smallpox and COVID-19. I have missed out on a few – people of my generation were born too early to be vaccinated against measles, mumps, rubella, chickenpox, rotavirus or human papillomavirus. I get a flu vaccine every year, and soon I will be old enough to be vaccinated against pneumococcal disease and shingles. All thanks to Sarah, the beautiful milkmaid.

The name of Edward Jenner lives on in the Jenner Institute, created in 2005 in Oxford, as a network of scientists to advance the science of vaccines. I was on the board of the Jenner Institute for several years and saw it grow into the "Silicon Valley" of vaccine research. Jenner investigators are working on vaccines for a host of diseases, including malaria, tuberculosis, Ebola and

COVID-19. Professor Sarah Gilbert, who led the work on the Oxford/AstraZeneca COVID-19 vaccine, is a Jenner investigator.

The story of smallpox vaccination is celebrated in the Edward Jenner Museum in Berkeley, Gloucestershire. On my visit there I learned about Jenner's life, his family, and how he died. I saw the simple thatched hut where he performed his vaccinations. In the gift shop I bought a print of the Chantry, the rather grand house where he lived. But for Sarah, all that exists is a print of her hand, with the blisters that were the source of Jenner's vaccine. She is simply "Case Number Sixteen" in his paper. The print of Sarah's hand has been reproduced on the cover of this book. With the help of the museum, I tracked down Michael Nelmes, her great, great, great, great grandson, who lives in Canberra, Australia. I learned that Sarah had six children and she died in 1840. She kept her perfect alabaster skin, thanks to the protection she received from her cow, Blossom. But that's all. Blossom has fared rather better; her hide hangs on the wall of the St Georges Medical School Library, in London, where Jenner completed his medical training. I've mentioned some of the heroes of vaccination: Jenner, Pasteur, Salk. There are just as many unsung heroes; Sarah is one of them.

3

The Invisible Army

In the length of time it takes to read this sentence, 943 people will have received a vaccine somewhere in the world (OK, maybe not so many for you super-fast readers). That's 5 billion doses a year (and that's not counting the COVID-19 vaccine roll out: over 11 billion doses and counting). No other prescription medicine comes close to vaccines. Vaccines are the only truly universal medical intervention. They are given in every continent, country, region, city, town and village in the world. Babies, schoolchildren, expectant mothers, travellers, workers, grandparents and presidents all get vaccinated. Queen Elizabeth II got her COVID-19 jab (and urged others to do the same). Fighting armies put down their weapons for a day to allow vaccination campaigns to go ahead.

The Oxford English Dictionary defines a vaccine as "an antigenic preparation used to stimulate the production of antibodies and provide immunity against disease". That's a bit of a mouthful but it's actually beautifully simple. The principle behind a vaccine hasn't changed since Edward Jenner's discovery. Take whatever it is that causes an infectious disease (known as the pathogen), modify it so that it can't cause the disease, but still makes you immune, then wait for the body to recognise it and mount an immune response. There are many ways of modifying the pathogen but the end game is always the same – trick your body into thinking it is fighting the real disease.

The part of the pathogen that the immune system recognises is known as the antigen. The antigens in vaccines are derived from either bacteria or viruses (apart from the malaria vaccine, which contains antigen derived from a single-celled parasite, called plasmodium). Come and meet these amazing invisible creatures.

Bacteria are single-celled, living organisms. They are tiny. Measuring between one and ten micrometres (millionths of a metre) across, they are only visible under a microscope. In comparison, human hair is between 17 and 180 micrometres thick. Bacteria can replicate themselves every twenty minutes, and have adapted to live in almost any environment. They have been found thriving in radioactive waste, boiling hot acid springs and deep in the earth's crust. One gram of soil from your garden contains 40 million bacteria. The total weight of all the bacteria on planet earth exceeds the weight of all the animals (including humans). Our bodies are teeming with bacteria. We have 37 trillion of them, the same as the total number of cells in our body. If you were to lay all the bacteria in your body, side by side, they would stretch around the circumference of the earth. Your gut alone contains up to a thousand different species of bacteria. Most of these are harmless passengers and some are actually very helpful. We couldn't live without the bacteria that inhabit our gut, helping us digest our food. The bacteria that inhabit our gut are collectively called our microbiome. A poorly functioning gut microbiome makes us prone to obesity, inflammatory bowel disease, and autoimmune diseases of the bowel. A bacterium that attacks its host is thankfully a rare event. Tuberculosis, whooping cough, diphtheria and tetanus are all examples of infections caused by bacteria that have decided to turn nasty.

DOI: 10.1201/9781003303879-3

Viruses are a very different ballgame. Even more abundant than bacteria, they are much, much smaller, measured in nanometres (billionths of a metre). To see a virus, you need a high-resolution microscope called an electron microscope. The electron microscope wasn't invented until 1931, which is one of the reasons that vaccines for viral diseases like influenza came later than for bacterial diseases. Viruses are hardy to say the least. In the 1990s, a team of scientists exhumed a body of an Inuit woman in the permafrost of a remote village in Alaska. She had died of influenza during the 1918 pandemic. Seventy-five years later, they were able to revive the genetic material of the virus in her body, enabling them to recreate its entire genetic sequence. In 2016, researchers from McMaster University in Ontario, Canada, were able to recover genetic material of the smallpox virus from a mummified boy who had been buried in Lithuania in the seventeenth century. The genetic material in these ancient corpses was not able to replicate, so it wasn't infectious. In the right conditions, however, some viruses can survive intact for many years and cause disease. Samples of smallpox virus have been found alive and well, stored in envelopes in laboratories for up to seven years. Unlike the fragments of viruses found in Alaska and Lithuania, these were capable of being infectious, which is one of the reasons why the destruction of laboratory stocks of smallpox virus was so critical to the eradication of the disease.

What really sets viruses apart from other microscopic invaders, however, is their ability to live inside the cells of another living being. In fact, their very existence depends on this, as they can only multiply when they are inside a cell. Some scientists don't even think of them as living organisms (especially bacteriologists, who spend their lives studying bacteria and tend to consider them as rather superior organisms). Viruses (their name in Latin means poison) can exhibit extremely antisocial behaviour. They force the cells of their host to make copies of themselves, often killing the cell in the process. Many viruses are harmless; however, they are generally rather unwelcome house guests. Polio, measles, Ebola, the common cold and of course COVID-19 all belong to the virus club.

When you encounter one of these microscopic creatures, there is a sequence of events that starts at the site where the initial invasion takes place. Although the infection has started, you do not develop symptoms right away. There is a period of time between getting infected and falling sick. This is the incubation period, and it's sometimes surprisingly long. Measles has an incubation period of seven to eighteen days, chickenpox can take more than three weeks to appear, and rabies symptoms can appear years after the bite of a rabid dog. Although you don't have symptoms during the incubation period, you can infect other people, especially just before you get symptoms. In some diseases, you are at your most infectious during the incubation period. As your body starts to fight the infection, you become less infectious to others, and eventually you clear it all together. Some infections, however, have the ability to persist in your body. Viruses are particularly good at this. They either become long-term chronic infections (like hepatitis B) or may become dormant (this is called latency) only to reappear many years later. This is what happens with the virus that causes chickenpox: after the initial infection, the virus lies dormant in nerve cells. Later in life, as your immune system ages, the virus comes back to life, this time causing shingles. Other viruses, like HIV, start very slowly, then become progressively more disruptive over time. They can also have long-term effects, like post-viral fatigue. Long COVID has already been recognised; it will take many years to determine all the long-term consequences. Viruses deserve serious respect.

These tiny organisms live in a delicate balance between the hosts they infect (us humans), and the environment that we both inhabit. A change in our behaviour or health status, or in the natural environment, can have a dramatic effect on the ability of a virus or bacterium to make us ill and infect others. The explosion in travel over the last fifty years has made it very easy for these microscopic passengers to hitch a ride to unlimited destinations, free of charge, no passport or visa required. Our ageing population is a great opportunity for the invisible army to take advantage of weakened immune systems. Age, sex, ethnic background, lifestyle, underlying disease and even your psychological state all affect both the likelihood of exposure to an infectious disease and the outcome if you catch it. The environment is no less important. Global warming means that disease-carrying insects can survive in new climates. The Asian Tiger mosquito, *Aedes albopictus*, is now firmly ensconced in the South of France. The mosquito first arrived in Europe in the late 1970s on ships carrying goods (they survived particularly well inside car tyres), slowly but surely establishing itself. This is the carrier of dengue fever, a deadly tropical disease that can cause internal bleeding, until recently only seen in tropical zones of Asia, South America and Africa. A steady trickle of home-grown cases of dengue fever has been reported in France over the last ten years, and this looks set to increase. The sandfly that carries leishmaniasis, another tropical disease, causing ulcers in skin and mucous membranes, has recently been found in Belgium and Germany. Warming temperatures in Canada have allowed the tick that bears Lyme disease to spread north. As climate change accelerates, we will see more infectious diseases spreading from tropical to temperate zones. Humans are also relentlessly pushing into new habitats, chopping down rainforests to make way for roads, industry, towns and farming. In Australia, this has forced the possum into closer contact with humans, carrying with them a flesh-eating bacterial disease, the Buruli ulcer. We are going to have many encounters with new foes.

The human body has a highly sophisticated immune system to deal with this army of invaders. We have some of it from birth (the innate immune system); the rest we learn as we go along (the adaptive immune system). The first lines of defence are physical and chemical barriers. Your skin, tears, the lining of your gut and lungs, the acid in your stomach are all designed to keep invaders at bay. Your body has a few tricks up its sleeve for ejecting unwanted visitors. Sneezing, coughing and vomiting are all highly effective methods for showing the door to uninvited gate crashers.

If the invader makes it past the first lines of defence, they encounter a much craftier response team. Your white blood cells (called leucocytes) are a highly disciplined and adaptable workforce. Leucocytes have evolved into different types, each with a specific function. Some swallow and destroy invaders without further ado, others instruct your body to produce antibodies. The job of this workforce is to give you immunity – your ability to protect yourself from infectious diseases. There are two arms of the immune system; antibodies and cells. Antibodies are produced by a specialised type of white blood cell known as a lymphocyte, specifically a B lymphocyte (or B cell). Antibodies have an arsenal of weapons which they use to deal with invaders. They can neutralise them with toxins, block them from getting into cells, and prevent them from multiplying. The cells involved in immunity are called T lymphocytes (T cells). They order the B cells to make antibodies and control the overall immune response. They also destroy cells that have been infected. The names T cell and B cell derive from where they were first discovered: T cells from the thymus gland (which sits behind your breastbone) and B cells from the Bursa of Fabricius, an organ found only in birds.

Your body also produces a host of chemicals that play a part in the immune response. These act as runners, ferrying information between cells and helping them do their work. The detection of a foreign invader triggers the production of a set of chemicals called cytokines, which mobilise the cells of the immune system. Another particularly helpful function of these chemicals is inflammation. The red, hot swelling under your skin, or in your throat, is caused by the expansion of tiny blood vessels, to accommodate the increased traffic that the immune response generates.

Like a disciplined army, your immune system has command posts where orders are carried out and immune cells report for duty. These are lymph nodes and are strategically positioned throughout your body. During an infection, as the defence mounts and cells report for duty, they swell up. The tender lump that you feel on the side of your neck when you have a throat infection is a lymph node, swarming with activity, like a hive of bees.

Vaccines work on the immune system in much the same way as invading bacteria and viruses. The immune system recognises a specific component in the vaccine, the antigen, and gets to work. Both T cells and B cells are involved in the response to a vaccine. Vaccines trigger an immune response, but not immediately. It takes time for the antigen to be recognised and processed by the immune system. Detectable antibodies usually start to appear seven to ten days after a vaccine is given. Sometimes the first attempt at antibody production is rather feeble, so you need to give a second or third vaccination. However, once you have decent antibody levels, you are in good shape. Your immune system has a spectacular memory. Some of your B cells – memory cells – are dedicated to committing information to a long-term memory bank. When it encounters the virus or bacterium, even after many years, the task force is quickly reassembled and swings into action immediately. There are also times when you need to jog the memory, by a booster vaccination; vaccine-induced immunological memory can be with you for life. It's more than thirty years since I was vaccinated against hepatitis A, and I am still protected. A certificate of vaccination against yellow fever is valid for life, thanks to immunological memory.

It's a very different story for those of us that don't have a properly functioning immune system. Some children are born with immune deficiency, and face a lifetime of recurrent infections. Others become immune deficient when they develop diseases like HIV or leukaemia, or become malnourished (this is one of the reasons infectious diseases exert such a dreadful toll in poor countries). Some drugs reduce the functioning of our immune system, such as chemotherapy for cancer treatment, and steroids in high doses. Immune deficiency is a double whammy. Not only are people with malfunctioning immune systems more susceptible to infectious disease, but they also don't respond as well to vaccines. Even worse, there are some types of vaccines that cannot be given to people with more serious immune deficiencies. These people rely on others being vaccinated for their protection.

Newborn babies are in a particularly perilous situation. They do inherit some immunity from their mother, either in the womb, with antibodies being ferried across the placenta, or from breast milk. This borrowed immunity (called passive immunity) is only a temporary loan and they have to quickly develop their own defences. Even in the wealthiest of societies, infection is a major killer of newborn babies. Ideally, all vaccines would be given at birth, or better still in the womb. Unfortunately, a baby's evolving immune system is not quite mature enough to be able to mount a strong response right away, which is why vaccinations usually start at six to eight weeks of age, although some (for example, the vaccine for tuberculosis) can be given at birth. One way of protecting the newborn is to vaccinate the mother during pregnancy. This is already recommended for influenza and whooping cough vaccines, and more recently for COVID-19. As more evidence on the safety of vaccination in pregnancy becomes available, further vaccines will likely be given to pregnant women in the future, both to protect mothers and their unborn children.

The delicate balance between infectious diseases, humans and the environment has shaped the course of human history. The advent of vaccines has enabled us to take some control over our destiny. The invisible army is still to be feared, but can be tamed.

4

Taming the Enemy

Vaccines work by tricking your immune system into thinking it is fighting a full-blown infection. Pulling off this con requires manipulation of the infectious agent, i.e., the bacterium or virus. The manipulation must disable the agent so that it doesn't make you sick, while preserving its ability to stimulate your immune system so you are protected. There are several ways this can be done, and they have become increasingly sophisticated. The two traditional methods were inactivation and attenuation or weakening. Later, only fragments of the virus or bacteria were used; the most modern vaccines now use only the genetic material of the infectious agent.

An inactivated vaccine is made by killing the virus or bacterium, either chemically or with heat. The virus or bacterium in an inactivated vaccine is dead, incapable of multiplying, also known as non-replicating. Many of the early vaccines of the nineteenth century such as rabies, typhoid and cholera were made by inactivation, and a few modern vaccines such as polio and hepatitis A still use this method. Their inability to multiply makes them very safe; however, they tend to provide protection which doesn't last for long, so booster injections have to be given. Inactivated polio vaccines need three initial doses, followed by two boosters, to provide full protection. This protection lasts for ten years, so if you travel somewhere that there is still polio and it is more than ten years since your last vaccination, you will need a further booster.

There is another type of non-replicating vaccine, known as a toxoid. There are two toxoid vaccines – diphtheria and tetanus. The symptoms of these diseases are not caused by the bacterium itself, but by the powerful toxin that they generate. The vaccine is made from the toxin, rather than bacterium itself. The toxin is inactivated, so that it can no longer cause disease. Like inactivated vaccines, toxoid vaccines cannot multiply, and usually require repeat boosters to maintain immunity. I have had no fewer than eight doses of tetanus toxoid vaccine in my life. This lifetime achievement is only exceeded by another inactivated vaccine, typhoid (which I've had twelve times).

The other classical type of vaccine is attenuated. The aim with this approach is not to kill the virus or bacteria, but to render it harmless. This is done by repeatedly growing it in an unnatural environment. In the natural world, viruses and bacteria are continually infecting different animal species and humans. To survive this continually changing environment, they have to adapt in order to survive. The less adaptable ones will lose out to those who can jump from species to species at will. This selection pressure is what allows them to retain their ability to infect you and make you ill. If you remove the selection pressure by growing them over and over and over again in the same environment, they will eventually lose their ability to cause disease. The environment used for this repeated growth is usually a specific type of cell. It can take up to 200 repeat cell cultures to sufficiently weaken the virus or bacterium so that it cannot cause disease.

These attenuated vaccines (often referred to as live attenuated vaccines or replicating vaccines) have a number of advantages over inactivated vaccines. Because they are alive, they grow and multiply in your body. This means your immune system gets a continuous stimulus over several days or even weeks. Live attenuated vaccines provide stronger, and longer-lasting

DOI: 10.1201/9781003303879-4

immunity than killed ones. Yellow fever is a live attenuated vaccine; a single dose will protect you for life. There are some downsides, however. The ability of live vaccines to multiply means that they can produce symptoms of the disease, albeit a much milder version. Measles vaccine is a good example. It's quite common for a child to develop a rash and mild fever about a week after the vaccine; a "mini measles". Very rarely, a live vaccine can produce a full-blown version of the disease. Paralysis following live polio vaccination (the version that is given by mouth) occurs at a rate of about one per 2 million doses. This is still much better than the actual disease, where up to one in ten people who are infected will get paralysis, however, it is one of the reasons why most polio vaccines given nowadays are the killed version, which cannot cause paralysis. Another drawback of live vaccines is that they cannot be given to people with severely weakened immune systems, as they may not be able to control the replication of the organism. Examples of live attenuated vaccines include measles, mumps, rubella, yellow fever, BCG (for tuberculosis) and oral polio vaccine.

A more refined approach to making vaccines started in the 1970s. Rather than using the entire virus or bacterium, only the part that generates the immune response, the antigen, was put in the vaccine. These are called subunit vaccines. Modern whooping cough vaccines are an example, containing between three and five purified components of the bacterium that causes whooping cough. In contrast, the early whooping cough vaccines used the entire bacterium, which has over 3,000 components. The advantage of including only the essential components is that side effects are less common. The trade-off is that they may not be so effective. It's a balancing act between reducing the amount of material in the vaccine without losing effectiveness.

For some vaccines, it's a particularly challenging balancing act. The bacteria that cause some types of meningitis are covered in a thick mucus-like coat called a polysaccharide. This polysaccharide coat is the bit that determines their ability to make you ill, so it needs to be in the vaccine; however, our immune system doesn't mount such a strong response to a polysaccharide as it does to other parts of the bacteria, which are made of protein. To get a round this, the polysaccharide is linked to a different protein, which helps it to stimulate the immune system, thus improving the immune response. These hybrid vaccines that contain polysaccharide joined to a protein are known as conjugates. Vaccines for meningococcal meningitis, pneumococcal disease (which causes pneumonia and blood poisoning), and *Haemophilus influenzae* type B ("Hib", another cause of meningitis) have been made using conjugate technologically. I have a personal research interest in this class of vaccines and conducted trials of several vaccines that ultimately ended up being used to vaccinate children against meningococcal meningitis and Hib, including one vaccine that combined both into one vaccine.

The latest, state of the art vaccines are made using various gene-based techniques. The first genetically engineered vaccine was hepatitis B. The genetic material – DNA (short for deoxyribonucleic acid) – of the hepatitis B virus is inserted into a harmless host organism: in this instance, *Saccharomyces cerevisiae*, better known as baker's yeast. The gene then instructs the host organism (called the vector) to start making the part of the hepatitis B virus that your immune system can recognise. Vaccines against human papillomavirus (HPV), the cause of cervical cancer, have been made using the same principle.

Hepatitis B and HPV vaccines both use genetic technology, but there is no genetic material in the final product. The last decade has seen huge advances with the development of vaccines that actually contain genetic material. There are two types – based on either DNA or RNA (ribonucleic acid). DNA is a bit like a brain. It has the knowledge to produce proteins – the building blocks of life – but lacks the physical ability to carry out its instructions. This is the job of messenger RNA or mRNA for short, the arms and legs of our genes. The DNA of someone with blue eyes has the code to produce cells with the right pigment, but it needs their RNA to execute production.

DNA vaccines contain the genetic material that has the code for the antigen of the vaccine, the part that stimulates an immune response. A DNA vaccine is either inserted into the gene of a harmless virus before injection or injected directly. Vaccines that use a harmless virus as the carrier for the genetic material are called viral vector vaccines. The genetic material for the virus is inserted into the harmless virus, which acts as a vector (the medical term for a carrier). The viral vector may sometimes replicate, but does not cause disease. Several of the COVID-19 vaccines are viral vector vaccines, including the one developed at Oxford University with AstraZeneca, the Johnson & Johnson vaccine, and my favourite – simply because of its name – Sputnik V. These COVID-19 vaccines use an adenovirus, one of the causes of the common cold, as the vector to carry the genetic information in the vaccine. A useful feature of viral vector vaccines is that the same vector can be used to make different vaccines. The adenovirus vector that is used for Johnson & Johnson's COVID-19 vaccine had already been used to make a highly effective Ebola vaccine a few years earlier.

Other types of DNA vaccines work by injecting the genetic material directly into the body (somewhat saucily known as naked DNA vaccines). The DNA is taken up by the body's cells and starts doing what DNA does – instructing the cells to produce the antigen. The vaccine is literally being manufactured inside your body. There are some naked DNA vaccines approved for use in animals, but research in humans is still at an early stage. This approach has been tried for several virus infections, including HIV, Zika virus and hepatitis B and some COVID-19 vaccines that are still in development.

All DNA-based vaccines produce a wide range of immune responses. They are stable, and have the big advantage of being relatively easy to produce in large amounts.

The second type of genetic vaccine is based on mRNA, the messenger of DNA. When injected, mRNA vaccines directly instruct the body to make antigen. Unlike DNA, RNA is unstable and gets broken down by your body soon after being injected. To prevent this from happening too quickly, it needs to be protected with something (often a lipid, which is a type of fat) before being injected. Even with this protective coat, the RNA only lasts a few hours, so it's a race against time to make the antigen. Some types of mRNA vaccines use a trick of modifying the RNA so that it is able to multiply inside the cell, known as self-amplifying messenger RNA or SAM for short. Like DNA vaccines, mRNA vaccines produce a broad range of immune responses but are even easier to manufacture. Two of the earliest approved COVID-19 vaccines, from Pfizer/BioNTech and Moderna, are mRNA-based.

Gene-based vaccines have several advantages over more traditional approaches. They can be developed quickly, as they don't need a lengthy process of cultivation and harvesting. As soon as the gene sequence of a virus is known, a vaccine can be constructed within days. This is one of the factors that enabled COVID-19 vaccines to be developed so quickly. They also have a big advantage in that they can be produced relatively easily in large quantities. This is obviously crucial in a pandemic.

There is a rather clever trick that is used to improve the immune response to some vaccines. Adjuvants (from the Latin *adjuvare*: to add) are naturally occurring substances that on their own have no effect on the immune system. However, when added to a vaccine, they boost its effect, tricking the immune system into mounting a more effective response. They improve the efficiency of the vaccine, rather like oil additives are used to improve engine efficiency. Adjuvants have several benefits. The immune response to an adjuvanted vaccine starts more quickly, so you are protected sooner. The level of immunity is higher, so the ability of an adjuvanted vaccine to protect you against the disease is often greater than a non-adjuvanted version. The protection last longer, so fewer booster doses are needed. "Faster, stronger, longer" was the slogan for one adjuvanted vaccine. Improving the immune response is particularly helpful for non-replicating vaccines, especially the more modern subunit ones that only have fragments of the bacterium or virus and need a helping hand.

The first adjuvants were aluminium salts. In the 1930s, they were used to improve the response to diphtheria and tetanus toxoids. Many vaccines in use today still contain aluminium hydroxide or aluminium phosphate – diphtheria, tetanus, whooping cough, hepatitis A and B to name a few. Some people have raised concerns about the safety of aluminium-containing vaccines. Aluminium is the most common metal in the earth's crust, and we are exposed to it all the time. Most foods, drinking water and breast milk contain aluminium. The amount of aluminium in vaccines is considerably less than we consume on a daily basis.

In recent years, many new adjuvants have been made from naturally occurring products, such as animal oils and plant derivatives.

The increasing use of adjuvants has raised further concerns about their safety. Adjuvanted vaccines do increase the risk of common side effects such as pain, swelling, fever. This is a small price to pay. There have been claims that adjuvants can cause more serious side effects; however, to date there is no scientific evidence to justify this. They are likely to feature in many of the new vaccines in development.

As the number of new vaccines increased, it posed a dilemma. How do you vaccinate people against so many diseases, particularly when they have to be given early in life? At one stage the US vaccination schedule demanded that babies get up to five injections in one visit. The answer was to develop combination vaccines that protect against more than one disease, with several vaccines in the same syringe, reducing the number of injections required. One of the most common combinations given to babies protects against six diseases – diphtheria, tetanus, whooping cough, polio, hepatitis B and *Haemophilus influenzae* type b. Another well-known combination vaccine is MMR – measles, mumps and rubella. There is theoretically no limit to the number of vaccines that can be combined in one syringe. The rate limiting factor is that the components sometimes interfere with each other, reducing the immune response. They can also cause more side effects. I once worked on a vaccine that was designed to protect against seven diseases. We ran trials of many different versions, but each time one of the components wouldn't produce a good enough immune response. Increasing the dose of that component would then reduce the response of one of the others. That vaccine was eventually abandoned. Despite the occasional set back, however, combinations are here to stay, and there will be more – a combined flu/COVID-19 vaccine is a likely candidate.

Most vaccines are given by injection; however, a few can be given in other ways. The two main non-injection routes are swallowed (oral) or squirted up the nose (intranasal). Instead of the immune response starting at the injection site, this time the first-line troops are mobilised in the lining of the gut (for an oral vaccine) or the membranes of the nose and throat (for an intranasal vaccine). In order for this to happen, the vaccine has to be able to grow in the cells that line the gut or nose and throat, so these vaccines are all of the live attenuated variety – a killed vaccine would not be able to grow.

There have been many attempts at making vaccines that can be given by mouth. The problem is that the vaccine has to get past the very hostile environment of your gut – which has acids, enzymes and other defence mechanisms – before it can reach the immune system. The result is that the immune system does not get a big enough stimulus to produce protective antibodies. The vaccine has to compete with all the other bacteria and viruses that inhabit your gut, which can sometimes reduce its ability to grow in it. If you have diarrhoea or vomiting, the vaccine does not even get a chance to get to the immune system. The most widely used oral vaccine is polio; there are also oral vaccines for typhoid fever, cholera and rotavirus, a common cause of childhood diarrhoea.

Vaccines given by nasal spray also have a hard time getting to your immune system. Your nasal passages are thick with tiny thin hairs, called cilia, that act like permanent cleaners, sweeping away unwanted visitors. When you have a cold, the lining of your nose responds by creating thick sticky mucus (better known as snot), barring the entry route for a vaccine. Sneezing blows away any vaccine that has managed to get past the mucus.

Intranasal vaccines are still relatively new. The only successful nasal spray vaccine to date is for the flu. When it is squirted up your nose, the flu virus in the vaccine attaches itself to the lining of the nose and throat. It starts to multiply, generating an immune response and triggering the chain of events that protect you against the strains of flu in the vaccine. Many vaccines in development are trying the same approach, and I expect we will see more intranasal vaccines over the next few years.

A brief mention of homeopathic vaccines: some people prefer these to conventional ones. Homeopathic vaccines are made from specimens of people or animals that have a disease. For example, a homeopathic rabies vaccine is made from the saliva of a rabid skunk. The specimen is diluted with water and given by mouth. There have been umpteen studies on their effectiveness, none of which have shown any benefit. The level of dilution makes any active ingredient almost non-existent. Most practicing homeopaths do not recommend these vaccines.

Vaccines have come a long way since Sarah Nelmes donated her cowpox for Jenner's vaccine. Many challenges remain. Despite more than thirty years of research, there is still no effective vaccine for HIV. Vaccines for the two other big killers – tuberculosis and malaria – do not provide full protection. There are no vaccines for herpes simplex, or most sexually transmitted diseases. New diseases will emerge, and it's only a question of when the next pandemic will strike. The COVID-19 pandemic has turned the world of vaccines upside down, turbo-charging research into new ways of developing and manufacturing vaccines. We are entering the second golden era of vaccination.

5

I'd Rather Be Jabbed Than Shot

I spent a year working as a community paediatrician in South East London. I would travel to clinics in Bermondsey, Lewisham, New Cross, Deptford and Rotherhithe. It was 1981, unemployment in the UK had just reached 3 million, and social deprivation was rife. My job was to check on the development of babies and young children, and vaccinate them against infectious diseases. Injecting a baby with a vaccine is simple. The more challenging – and interesting – part of the job was the conversations I had with parents about their concerns. I didn't have any children at the time, but years later when my two-month-old daughter had her first vaccination, I can't deny that I felt a tad anxious. The prospect of sticking a needle into a perfectly healthy baby is surely enough to make the most rational parent ask questions. Not surprisingly, the fact that the vaccine had to be given by injection was a big issue for many parents. Almost daily, someone would ask why their baby had to have "the needle". I tried different approaches to tackle this anxiety. "We do vaccinations here all the time, nothing to worry about" (patronising); "You need to do this for your baby's health" (scare mongering); "Your baby will hardly feel anything" (a bit of an exaggeration and not convincing); however, some parents were simply not prepared to let their children be injected with a needle. I ended up running a specialist clinic for parents that had major concerns about having their children vaccinated, where I was able to devote more time to talk through their concerns. Once a week I would drive round the North Circular to a rather drab-looking health centre in Redbridge, where I spent the day talking to parents about the reasons they were hesitant to get their child vaccinated. There were a few common themes – my child is allergic to eggs (some vaccines are grown on cells derived from chicks), there's a family history of fits, I had reactions to vaccines myself as a child. Being able to discuss their concerns, explain how vaccines work and their side effects, usually resulted in the parent deciding to go ahead. Sometimes this only happened after two or three consultations. My experience at the Redbridge clinic really helped my understanding of parents' anxieties about vaccines. I was struck by the fact that every discussion was about a vaccine that was given by injection. No-one ever asked me about the polio vaccine, which at the time was given by mouth. Not once – although, paradoxically, that is the one vaccine for which there is a known serious (but fortunately rare) side effect: paralysis. The bottom line is that people do not like needles. Fear of needles – needle phobia – is a recognised medical condition. It's estimated that up to ten percent of people suffer from needle phobia. I used to run a research programme at Nottingham University. Once a year I would take a blood sample from all the first-year medical students, to measure their antibodies. Without fail, someone would faint at the prospect of me sticking a needle in their arm (typically it would be a strapping, rugby-playing male who keeled over). Needles put people off getting vaccinated; removing them would be a game changer for vaccination.

There has been no shortage of effort to develop needle-free vaccines. Researchers, vaccine companies and governments have all tried very hard to discover alternatives. They have tried nasal sprays, skin patches, tiny needles that you can't feel, and edible vaccines. Someone even

DOI: 10.1201/9781003303879-5

came up with the idea of using genetically modified bananas to give vaccines (it didn't work). There have been some successes, but most vaccines today still have to be given by injection.

For a vaccine to work, it has to reach your body's immune system. The most efficient way to get a vaccine in contact with your body's immune system is to inject it into a muscle. Your muscles are teeming with the various types of cells that make up your immune system. When you inject a vaccine into a muscle, it quickly meets these cells. They recognise the vaccine and start instructing your body to make antibodies that will allow you to fight off infections in the future. There are a few oral vaccines and one which can be given as a nasal spray, but intramuscular injection is the best route for most vaccines (an exception is BCG, the vaccine for tuberculosis, which is injected into the skin).

Giving a vaccine by injection is pretty straightforward. You need a syringe, a needle and of course the vaccine. The syringe has two parts – the barrel containing the vaccine, and the plunger, which pushes the vaccine from the barrel through the needle and into the muscle. The needle is attached to the barrel of the syringe before giving the injection. Some syringes are made with the needle pre-attached. The vaccine is drawn up into the syringe from a small bottle (called a vial) using the needle. Sometimes it is a powder that has to first be dissolved before being drawn up. To make life easier, some manufacturers have already put the vaccine in the syringe beforehand – these are called pre-filled syringes. The vaccine is now ready to be injected into a muscle. The best place to give the injection is where there is a decent-sized muscle, which is easy to access. In adults and older children, this is the upper part of the arm, and in babies the thigh is the best spot. The needle is pushed through the skin, usually at a right angle, and the vaccine is injected. The amount of vaccine that is usually injected is 0.5 ml. This is equivalent to one-tenth of a standard teaspoon. The whole procedure takes a few seconds.

Several people have tried to measure the amount of pain caused by a vaccination. This is difficult, because our perception of pain is clouded by how painful we think something is going to be. One way to get an unbiased assessment of vaccination pain is to measure it in babies and very young children. They have not yet developed any opinions about injections, or how painful they are going to be. They cannot verbally express how much pain they feel; however, there are several techniques to measure pain in very young children, for example by changes in their facial expressions. Several studies have been conducted in babies and young children to measure the amount of pain felt immediately after vaccination. The results varied depending on which vaccine was given, but in all the studies the level of pain was mild and short-lived. Vaccine injections really don't hurt that much.

The problem is that the fear of injections goes beyond the actual pain they cause. Injections are given with needles, and we associate needles with pain. Needles have negative connotations. They are the tools of recreational drug users, discarded in parks. They have caused outbreaks of hepatitis and AIDS. They look scary, particularly when exaggerated in cartoons and the popular press. Anti-vaccine protestors carry banners displaying needles the size of javelins. We use negative language to describe injections. "Kids Killer Diseases Face Big Jabs Blitz", screamed the headline of a tabloid, announcing the launch of the measles/mumps/rubella vaccine in the UK. Who wants to give their baby a Big Jab, especially during a Blitz? JABS (Justice, Awareness and Basic Support) is the name of a prominent anti-vaccination group. In my native Scotland, vaccinations are called jags, the same word used to describe the sharp painful thorns of the national emblem, the thistle. Americans call them shots. Yes, shots! Is a needle in the same category as a gun? One of the first anti-vaccine books was called *DTP – A Shot in the Dark*, re-enforcing the negative stereotype. A few years ago, I went to an international vaccine conference. On the final day, I was chairing a lively debate on why vaccination uptake rates were falling around the world. Predictably, the delegates started to berate the lack of progress in needle-free vaccination as a big swing factor. At one point, an American woman stood up and said that it didn't help that vaccines were referred to as jabs in the UK. In response, Jeffrey Almond, the head of research at the French vaccine company, Sanofi Pasteur, pointed out that in the United States they were called shots. Jeffrey is a down-to-earth Northerner with a very dry sense of humour. "Mr Chairman, I'd rather be jabbed than shot," he quipped.

Since it looks like giving vaccines by injection will be around for a while, there are few useful tips to reduce the discomfort. Good technique helps. Injections are less painful if they are given quickly but not too forcefully.

There are local anaesthetic creams that can be rubbed into the skin beforehand. Provided this is done in good time (at least one hour before the injection), it is pretty effective at dulling the pain. In babies, breastfeeding during and immediately after vaccination has been shown to reduce the amount of crying after the injection. Other distractions (toys, videos, etc.) are good for babies, but don't work for cynical older children. It's quite common for parents to give their baby a painkiller such as paracetamol, before getting a vaccine. This may reduce the risk of side effects such as fever, but doesn't actually reduce the pain at the time of the injection. It can also interfere with the immune response of the vaccine, so it's best to use painkillers only if there is reaction to the vaccine. Some people believe that rubbing the skin after the injection helps dull the pain, as the rubbing sensation distracts your brain from the pain, but this is probably a waste of time.

Needles and syringes have improved beyond recognition since the first hypodermic syringe was invented in 1853 by a Scotsman, Alexander Wood (a Frenchman, Charles Pravaz, invented something similar at around the same time, but it was Wood's version that became the standard). He used his device to inject an eighty-year-old woman suffering from myalgia (muscle pain) with morphine dissolved in sherry. She fell into a deep sleep but when she regained consciousness, she was free from pain. Please don't try this at home. One of the biggest advances in vaccination was the use of disposable syringes, so that after the vaccine is given, the needle does not need to be re-used. This avoids transmitting diseases like hepatitis and HIV, although the World Health Organization estimates that even today, millions of infections are caused by re-use of syringes. Vaccinations in the developing world are often given with syringes that automatically lock after use, preventing them from being re-used. Several features of needles have been improved to make them less painful – increasing their sharpness with more sophisticated techniques to grind the tip of the needle to the smallest diameter, adding a thin layer of lubricant, and making the wall of the needle thinner without reducing the flow rate of the vaccine. Becton Dickinson, the biggest manufacturer of vaccine needles in the world (they produce 2 to 3 billion a year and many more since COVID), has an entire research division dedicated to improving the safety and feel of needles and syringes. The next generation of needles will be "microneedle" devices that have miniscule needles about the diameter of a human hair. Not only will these be less painful, but they also have the potential to improve the effectiveness of vaccines and could even be self-administered.

While we are waiting for someone to invent a needle-free vaccine we also need to de-stigmatise injections. Fear plays a big part in how people react to being vaccinated. Parents transmit this fear to their children. I saw this every day in my well baby clinics in London. When a smiling, calm parent would bring her baby for an injection, the baby's crying would be short-lived, if at all. The stressed parent who anxiously clutched their baby during the vaccination had the opposite effect. In my Redbridge clinic, where I had time to talk through the whole process, it helped dispel some of these anxieties and most babies didn't cry. Its ok to be jabbed. It's even ok to be shot.

6

The Long and Winding Road

Sixty-five! One hundred and ten! Eighty-four! Each dancer held a banner aloft, bearing a number. They whooped and cheered. The audience clapped, stamped their feet and started singing. It was party time. I got up and joined the dancers. I was brimming with excitement.

This was no ordinary disco. I was in the function room of the Hippo View Lodge in Liwonde, a remote part of southern Malawi. Outside there was a lake with a lopsided sign that read "Beware of the Crocodiles". The dancers were nurses, and the numbers on their banners represented the number of children they each had recruited to a trial of a vaccine against rotavirus. They had written the song they danced to. I have a recording of *The Ndirande* song; their soaring, joyous voices still give me goosebumps. Rotavirus is one of the main causes of diarrhoea in babies. In the Western world, most babies recover from rotavirus diarrhoea, but in Africa, it claims half a million infant deaths every year. When Bill Gates first heard about the number of rotavirus deaths, he said, "That can't be right. I read the news all the time. I read about plane crashes and freak accidents. Where is the news about these half-million kids dying?" I was working in the research department of GlaxoSmithKline, the vaccine company that sponsored the Malawi rotavirus vaccine trial, and was visiting Malawi to see how it was progressing. It was progressing well. The nurses had recruited 1,773 babies in the trial. This was enough to be able to determine whether the vaccine was effective. It had already been shown to work in other countries, but this was the first time it had been studied in Africa. The results of the trial were crucial in deciding whether the vaccine could be approved for use in developing countries, where the need was greatest. Most of the half-million deaths every year occurred there. The vaccine had to work in Africa, where babies are less well nourished, malaria is rife, and other types of diarrhoea might reduce the impact of the vaccine. What was needed was a trial, done in these exacting conditions, to the highest international standards. There could be no comprise on quality. This was non-negotiable. The trial had been audited twice before my visit. It passed with flying colours both times, and the auditors were so impressed with what they saw that they presented it at several conferences.

The Malawi rotavirus vaccine trial was an important milestone, but it was neither the beginning nor the end of the research programme. The first trials had started several years before my visit to Hippo Lodge in 2008. Twelve years after my visit, I contacted the two principal investigators of the Malawi rotavirus vaccine trial. They were still there, working on rotavirus vaccines, doing more trials (their latest research is on the effect of giving the vaccine at birth; it is usually given from six weeks of age).

Vaccine research is not for the faint-hearted. It typically takes between ten and fifteen years to take an experimental vaccine in a laboratory to the point where it can be approved for use, although this can be fast-tracked in an emergency (I'll talk about COVID-19 later). Developing a vaccine is a complex journey, that starts in the laboratory, then progresses through several phases of trials. It's a long, winding road, with many bumps along the way.

The first step is to decide which version of the vaccine is the most promising to be progressed. This is called candidate selection. The candidate is chosen based on what is already known about

DOI: 10.1201/9781003303879-6

the infectious disease. If a vaccine already exists, and the aim is to make a better one, this is easier than if it is for a completely new disease, although there may be helpful clues from similar diseases. This is one of the reasons that COVID-19 vaccines could be developed so quickly – vaccines were already undergoing trials for other pandemic diseases like Ebola, SARS (Severe Acute Respiratory Syndrome) and MERS (Middle East Respiratory Syndrome).

Sometimes more than one candidate is selected initially. The probability of success for a new vaccine, starting from scratch, is pretty low, so it's a good idea to have more than one horse in the race.

Once the candidate(s) are selected, tests are carried out to check, as far as possible, that the vaccine will be safe and have a good chance of working in humans. This is called the preclinical research phase, and it refers to all the stages that happen before studies start in humans.

In the preclinical phase, a whole range of chemical and physical tests are done to check that all the components of the vaccine are present in consistent amounts, there are no impurities, and they are stable. If it succeeds, the vaccine will eventually be mass-produced and given to millions of people, so the basic recipe has to be sound.

The preclinical phase also involves studies in animals. Some people oppose the use of animals in medical research. The lobby against animal research is particularly strong in the UK. In one incident, animal rights activists placed bombs under the cars of two researchers from a laboratory in Porton Down, near Salisbury. Luckily, no-one was seriously injured. The reality is that the best way to predict what will happen in a human is to try it in an animal. The use of animals in research is highly regulated, to ensure the minimum number of animals possible are used. The animals are kept in the best possible conditions, in highly specialised centres. Every animal experiment has to be approved by a regulatory agency. Scientists are continually looking for ways to reduce the number of animals in medical research.

The aim of these preclinical studies is to look for side effects and determine whether the vaccine can produce immune responses. The first animal studies are usually done in rats or mice. Later studies usually use larger animals, including monkeys. Several different doses will be tested to work out which is best to go forward into human studies. The safety of the vaccine is checked by looking for evidence of inflammation, effects on the immune system and the vital organs. Other studies look for the appearance of antibodies after vaccination, to provide clues on whether the vaccine will be effective. If these are promising, a so-called challenge study is often carried out. The animal is vaccinated, then exposed to the infectious disease to see if they are protected. This may sound unethical; however, a challenge study only involves a handful of animals, and because the information they generate is so useful, it avoids using larger numbers of animals in other less informative studies.

While these animal studies are helpful, they are not completely predictive. Something that generates an immune response in a mouse may not do the same in a human being. The absence of a side effect in an animal does not guarantee that it will be safe in humans.

When all the preclinical research is done, the next stage of the journey can begin – the clinical phase, with studies in humans for the first time. This a critical step in vaccine research, and is not taken lightly. The most important overriding principle in clinical research is the wellbeing of people who volunteer to take part in the studies. The principle of putting the wellbeing of study volunteers above all other considerations was first enshrined in 1964, in the Declaration of Helsinki. The Declaration puts a moral obligation on doctors all over the world to respect the rights of individuals in research. The Declaration has been backed up by legislation in most countries and there are established international standards for research, such as Good Clinical Practice (GCP). The regulatory authority of the country where a trial is being conducted will often visit the study site to check that the trial is being conducted to these standards. The research organisation or company that is running the trial will also carry out its own internal audits.

The first human trial is called, rather obviously, a "first-time-in-human" study. After my job in the research department of GlaxoSmithKline Vaccines, I went on to become the company's Chief Medical Officer. The Chief Medical Officer in a pharmaceutical company is there to ensure the highest ethical standards in research; the "voice of the patient". One of my responsibilities was to decide whether or not an experimental vaccine could have the green light for a first-time-in-human study. I had access to all the preclinical data, and a team of experts to advise me, but at some point, I would have to say yes or no. Saying no meant stopping, or at least delaying, the development of a vaccine that might save thousands of lives. Saying yes meant exposing volunteers to a vaccine for the first time. It was a balance of benefit and risk. Some decisions were easier than others. When an epidemic of Ebola broke out in West Africa, the need to start vaccine trials as quickly as possible was obvious, particularly as there was a wealth of reassuring preclinical data. A less obvious decision would be to start a trial with a vaccine that was an improvement on an existing version, which contained an adjuvant that would increase the number of side effects. Not all candidates got the go-ahead. I would always think about what I would do if someone in my family was going to volunteer for the trial. At this stage, no-one knows whether the vaccine is going to work, so I thought very carefully about what risks there might be to these early volunteers, and how to reduce these risks.

There are various ways to safeguard the safety of trial volunteers. First-time-in-human studies are done in healthy adults. Adults with underlying health conditions are excluded from these early studies, and there is often an upper age limit, typically around sixty. The vaccine may eventually be intended for children, or the elderly, but the safest way to test a vaccine for the first time is in a healthy adult. The number of people in a first-time-in-human trial is small – usually twenty to a hundred, and once I gave the go-ahead for a trial, I specified a maximum number of people per day that could be given the vaccine, with a big enough gap between each person getting vaccinated so that if someone did develop a severe reaction (a very rare event in a vaccine trial), it could be recognised, and the trial halted. First-time-in-human studies could only be done in centres where there was immediate access to an intensive care unit, so if someone did develop a severe reaction, they would have the best possible treatment. Centres that run first-time-in-human studies are state-of-the-art facilities, usually part of a large university hospital. They are staffed by people with extensive experience in these studies. I worked a lot with the centre at the University of Ghent in Belgium, where they have conducted over 250 vaccine trials. They understand how to run trials inside out and have all the facilities to treat anyone who develops a serious side effect.

A further safeguard in clinical trials is "holding rules" – if a certain number of people develop side effects, the trial is put on hold while they are investigated. Only when it has been established that the vaccine is not the cause, or that the side effect is not dangerous, can the trial resume. It is very uncommon for a vaccine trial to be halted permanently in a first-time-in-human study. It never happened in any trial I was involved with, although I paused studies on numerous occasions while investigations were carried out. This is common practice in clinical research and is all part of ensuring the safety of study participants.

All clinical trials have to be approved by an ethics committee. This is a group of people independent from the researchers. They include health professionals, but also often members of the public. There are established standards for the composition and functioning of ethics committees. They also have to be approved by the regulatory authority of the country where the trial is conducted. They scrutinise all aspects of trials to make sure that the volunteers have the best possible protection and there is no coercion.

Volunteers in trials at GlaxoSmithKline were not paid to take part in trials, although they could be compensated for any expenses or loss of earnings. This was an important principle for me and is widely applied by most researchers. Someone who volunteers for a trial to make money may be taking part in something they don't necessarily feel comfortable with.

Checking whether a vaccine is safe in a human involves a battery of tests and examinations. The most common side effects of vaccines are a mild fever and a local reaction at the injection site, with swelling, redness and sometimes pain. These side effects are all monitored regularly by study nurses. These study nurses are hired specifically for the trial and are highly trained to provide the best possible care for the study volunteers. Volunteers keep diaries to record any symptoms, and anything more serious is followed up to get a diagnosis and to determine whether it is related to the vaccine. Blood samples are taken at regular intervals. These are used to check whether the volunteer is developing immunity to the vaccine, by measuring antibody levels. The blood samples are also tested for various chemicals that are naturally present, such as sodium and potassium (electrolytes), and proteins that indicate whether the liver and kidneys are functioning properly. The different types of blood cells (red, white and platelets), and the level of haemoglobin, are also tested. An abnormal result may indicate a side effect and is followed up with further tests. Tests are also done on urine samples. The idea is to get as much information as possible about the safety of the vaccine, in the fewest number of people. No stone is left unturned. Later trials will be much bigger, eventually exposing thousands of people, so the more you can find out about any side effects at this stage, the better. Doing so many tests inevitably throws up abnormal results which might not be related to the vaccine. I recall one volunteer who had persistently high levels of protein in his urine. It turned out he was a fitness fanatic who exercised for several hours a day, a well-known cause of elevated protein in the urine.

Human challenge studies, where people are deliberately given an infectious disease after being vaccinated, are one way of getting information quickly about a vaccine. They have the huge advantage of being able to test the effectiveness of the vaccine without having to wait for a much larger trial. They are only done in specialised centres, under highly controlled conditions. The volunteers are monitored closely so they can be treated immediately if they become ill. They are kept in strict quarantine, with full protective equipment for the research team. A work colleague of mine once famously volunteered for a human challenge study for a malaria vaccine. After being given the experimental vaccine, he allowed infected mosquitos to feed on his arm. The vaccine didn't work, and he got a very unpleasant bout of malaria. Luckily, he lived to tell the tale, and went on to pioneer the development of the vaccine that is now approved and being rolled out in parts of Africa. As well as being a top vaccine researcher, he is an ace guitarist and singer. We played together in a rock band, called Dokter Rokter (groan).

There has been much debate about whether human challenge studies could have been done to speed up research on COVID-19 vaccines even further. The argument against doing these studies is that there isn't an effective treatment should a volunteer get sick. Others have argued that as long as volunteers fully understand the risks, then it is ethical do these studies. As treatment for COVID-19 has improved, the balance is shifting towards human challenge studies, and they are likely to feature in the development of the next generation of COVID-19 vaccines.

Once the first-time-in-human study is over, there may be other small trials to look at what happens with the same vaccine, but containing different amounts of the active ingredient. The idea is to see how volunteers react to different doses, to work out which is the best dose to take forward into larger trials. It's rather like trying different amounts of spices to make a perfect curry and is called dose ranging. Too low a dose and the vaccine won't generate antibodies. Too high a dose causes unacceptable side effects. The aim is to find the lowest possible dose that still generates antibodies. Surprisingly, there isn't necessarily a direct correlation between the dose and the response. In the trial of the Oxford/AstraZeneca COVID-19 vaccine, volunteers who received a half dose for their first injection were better protected than those who got the full dose.

These early studies are collectively called Phase 1 and usually take a few months. It is relatively uncommon for a vaccine trial to be stopped at this stage. Most new vaccines are made with technology that is tried and tested, so unpredictable side effects are less likely. If a vaccine fails in Phase 1, it is usually due to a low immune response, and this can often be rectified by giving a higher dose. This is rather different from the world of drug development, where compounds that work in novel ways are being discovered and tested all the time. The "probability of success" – the likelihood that a new compound progresses beyond Phase 1 – is higher for vaccines than it is for drugs. Vaccines are a relatively safe bet from a research point of view.

If a vaccine is successful in Phase 1, Phase 2 can begin. Here, the objective is different. The vaccine trials are not done in healthy adult volunteers, but in the people that you eventually want to benefit from the vaccine. This may be young children, teenagers, the elderly or people with specific medical conditions. In Phase 2, the goal is to show "proof of concept"; i.e. whether the vaccine is likely to be safe and effective in the population for whom it is eventually intended. Usually, the focus is on one "target" group – those that stand to benefit the most from the vaccine. I have worked on several types of meningitis vaccine over the years. The Phase 1 studies were done in adults, but the Phase 2 studies would have to be done in babies and teenagers, who would eventually be given the vaccine.

Phase 2 vaccine trials usually involve several hundred people. As in Phase 1 trials, trial volunteers keep symptom diary cards, with regular checks for fever and local reactions, and regular blood samples are taken. Study nurses keep in regular contact with the volunteers.

Phase 2 vaccine trials often involve young children for the first time. This raises an ethical dilemma. An eighteen-month-old baby cannot understand the implications of being in a trial, nor describe their symptoms. The parents have to decide whether they want their child to participate in the trial. They have to think about the benefits and the risks from their child's point of view. This applies to any research involving children; however, vaccine trials in children are rather unique. Children in vaccine trials are healthy, so the balance of benefit and risk is very different than in a drug trial. A parent enrolling their child in a trial for a new cancer treatment will probably accept the risk of a severe side effect in exchange for the possibility of a cure. The situation is very different in a vaccine trial. People who volunteer for vaccine trials are healthy. During the trial they will receive a vaccine. The vaccine might protect them against a future attack from the infectious disease but there is no immediate tangible benefit. A parent of a child in a vaccine trial is less likely to accept the risk of side effects from the experimental vaccine, for an uncertain, future benefit. This makes it more challenging to recruit children to vaccine trials compared to trials for drugs that might provide a cure.

Vaccines are often designed to protect against diseases which are most common in less developed countries. This means the research has to be done there. The world's first malaria vaccine was approved a few years ago after many years of clinical research. This was only possible because the trials were carried out in Africa, where there is enough malaria to show whether the vaccine could prevent it. Doing research in developing countries, especially in children, is fraught with difficulties. Parents in developing countries are often illiterate. They cannot read the lengthy informed consent forms that describe exactly what is in the vaccine, what is going to happen in the trial, and what side effects to expect. There are several ways to overcome this. In the Malawi rotavirus trial, we produced leaflets and posters with simple diagrams to explain what exactly would be involved in volunteering for the trial. A drawing of a thermometer was used to show how to take a baby's temperature, with the sun and moon indicating day or night-time readings. There were pictures of babies looking lethargic, unhappy and sleepy, to indicate their condition. The drawings of a bout of diarrhoea were a work of art. When a parent showed interest in the trial, we would arrange for someone she knew and trusted to explain all the procedures that take place. During the actual consent process, which would be done with a thumbprint, there would be an independent witness present. A video recording of the consent process is another way to ensure the volunteer fully understands the implications of joining the trial, and that they have the right to withdraw at any time, without giving a reason.

Another issue is that mothers in developing countries start having their babies much younger than in Europe or the United States. They are sometimes still children themselves. There has been a lot of debate about whether a mother, who is below the legal age of consent, can make decisions on behalf of her child. This became a big issue in a trial that I was involved in South America. We were testing a vaccine against pneumonia. Many of the mothers that wanted their babies to participate were underage, and sometimes the father was not involved in bringing up the child. The laws in the South American countries didn't really address the issue. We decided to come up with a set of guiding principles to help figure out how decide when it would be ok to recruit babies of young mothers to a trial and published a paper to help decision-making in this situation. Several things need to be taken into account: What is the capacity of a young mother to make rational decisions about participating in research? (It has been shown that the ability to make an informed decision is as good as an adult by twelve to fourteen years of age.) Would excluding young mothers, who are often vulnerable, from the opportunity of being in the trial, further disadvantage them? Are there local cultural factors that impact how young mothers are viewed in society? In some countries, very young mothers are the norm.

The informed consent process brings additional cultural challenges in developing countries. People do not have the same perception about health and disease and may not relate to western medicine. In Malawi, some parents believed that if you took a blood sample from a child, you were going to sell it to the witch doctor.

The aim of a Phase 2 trial programme is to show proof of concept. To do this for a vaccine, you need to show that people in the trial develop antibodies against the disease. You don't yet know whether these antibodies will actually protect people against the disease – that is the purpose of Phase 3 trials – but if you can show that antibodies increase after getting the vaccine, there is a reasonable expectation that it will work. There is usually more than one dose of vaccine tested in Phase 2. The one with the best antibody response, that has acceptable side effects, will be chosen to progress to Phase 3. Different schedules will also be tested – how many injections and whether to give a booster. The vaccine may also be tested in different age groups. This is also the time to try the vaccine in people who are at particular risk from the infectious disease, for example older people or those with underlying conditions. They may not respond as well to the vaccine, but they are the ones who are going to need it most. Phase 2 therefore involves multiple studies, often conducted in parallel. Side effects are measured in Phase 2, however, because there are only a few hundred people involved, only the most common side effects will be picked up. Something that happens after 1-per-1,000 vaccinations may not occur at all in Phase 2. Statisticians use a "rule of three" – to detect something that occurs 1 in 1,000 times, you need to study 3,000 people to have a good chance of detecting it. Much bigger numbers are required to detect rare side effects. A side effect that occurs in a Phase 2 study will need to be studied in more detail in Phase 3. And this is where the road gets longer, and considerably more winding.

Beware of the Crocodiles

The Malawi rotavirus Phase 3 trial was conducted in four centres in and around Blantyre: Ndirande, Limbe, Bangwe and Zingwangwa. Blantyre is the commercial hub of Malawi. Founded by Scottish missionaries, it lies in southern Malawi, close to Lilongwe National Park, home to buffalo, antelope, elephants, baboons, black rhinoceros, hippo, and is one of the best places in Africa to spot Nile crocodiles. Despite the warning sign, I didn't see any crocodiles during my stay at Hippo View Lodge (I didn't see any hippos either, but the mosquitos were spectacular).

Phase 3 is the definitive proof of whether a vaccine can protect against a disease. The word that is used to describe the extent to which a vaccine protects against a disease is efficacy. The efficacy of a vaccine is measured as the reduction in disease in people who get the vaccine compared to people who don't get it, in a situation where everybody is at risk of catching the disease.

The basic design of a Phase 3 trial is to recruit a group of people who will get the experimental vaccine and a group of people who will not receive the vaccine, known as the control group. The trial has to be done someplace where the disease is sufficiently common so that enough people will be exposed to the disease to see if there is a difference between the vaccinated group and the unvaccinated control group.

It is important that people do not know whether they have had the experimental vaccine or are in the control group. Knowing whether or not you have had a vaccine will inevitably bias your observations. You may be more likely to report side effects, and less likely to report symptoms of the disease, if you think you have had the vaccine. To avoid this bias, people in the unvaccinated control group are given something that looks exactly the same as the vaccine. This dummy vaccine is called a placebo (the name is from the Latin word which means "I shall be pleasing"). Sometimes the placebo will actually be another vaccine, which has been made to look like the experimental vaccine. The Phase 3 trial of the COVID-19 vaccine developed by Oxford University with AstraZeneca used a meningitis vaccine as the control. The advantage of this is that everyone in the trial has the opportunity to benefit, not just those that receive the experimental vaccine. Either you get the experimental vaccine, in which case you have the chance of being protected against the disease under investigation, in this case COVID-19, or you get the control vaccine, in which case you get protected against something else. The Oxford COVID-19 trial recruited adults who would not normally get vaccinated against meningitis, so those in the control group received a vaccine they would not otherwise have had.

Another important design feature of a Phase 3 trial is that neither the trial volunteer, or the person actually giving the vaccine, knows whether it is the experimental vaccine or the control. A nurse or a doctor is just as prone to biased observations as a participant in a trial. They will be more likely to report a side effect if they think it has occurred in someone who got the experimental vaccine than if it was someone who was given the placebo. For this reason, the experimental vaccine and the placebo need to look identical. Researchers go to great lengths to ensure that both the volunteers in a Phase 3 trial, and the health professionals who are conducting the

DOI: 10.1201/9781003303879-7

trial, are "blinded", so that no-one knows who has received the vaccine and who received the placebo. Everybody in the trial is assigned a number and there is a code which records which numbers correspond to people who got the vaccine versus those who got the control. People enrolled into a Phase 3 trial are randomly allocated by a computer-generated program, to be in the vaccine group or the placebo group. Only at the end of the trial is the code broken, so it can be revealed who was in which group.

This design is called a double-blind, randomised, placebo-controlled trial, and is the gold standard in research. It isn't always possible – usually for ethical reasons – to do a double-blind placebo-controlled trial. For example, if you wanted to test an improved version of an existing vaccine, you couldn't recruit volunteers to a trial in which they would not receive the existing vaccine if they ended up in the control group. In this situation trial volunteers would either get the existing vaccine or the improved one. There are alternative study designs for these situations but none are as free from bias as a double-blind, randomised, placebo-controlled trial.

Phase 3 vaccine trials usually involve several thousand volunteers, which is more than in drug trials. The reason is that in a vaccine trial, you are measuring the occurrence of a disease over time in people who do not have the disease at the start of the trial. If the disease is not very common, you need to recruit large numbers of people to show a difference in the subsequent rate of disease between the vaccinated and the non-vaccinated group. Pfizer's Phase 3 COVID-19 trial recruited more than 43,000 volunteers. In a drug trial, everyone already has the disease at the start of the trial, and you are looking to demonstrate a cure, or an improvement in symptoms. This requires fewer volunteers. A further complication with vaccine trials is that some diseases only occur at certain times of the year and are rather unpredictable. Flu is an example. You may have to follow the trial volunteers for more than one season to have enough cases. Before starting a Phase 3 trial, you need to know exactly how much disease is occurring, in order to plan how many volunteers you will need to recruit and how long it will take to obtain a meaningful result. It can take up to a year to establish this baseline. Planning a Phase 3 trial for a new disease like COVID-19 is even more of a headache, as no-one knows how the disease is going to evolve. As it turned out, many of the initial Phase 3 trials started recruiting just when the second wave of disease hit, so there was more disease than anticipated. The study volunteers were quickly exposed to the disease, and it soon became apparent that those who were in the vaccine group were protected.

One question that vexes vaccine researchers more than most is how to define the disease they are looking for. It sounds rather obvious – either you get the disease, or you don't – but it's a lot more complicated than that. Are you looking for all cases of the disease, including very mild ones, or do you just want to find the more serious ones? Do you need to have the diagnosis of all cases confirmed by laboratory tests? What about people who get the infection but have no symptoms? The effect of a vaccine will be different depending on how you define a case. Let's consider the design of a trial against whooping cough vaccine as an example. If you just look for cases in which they had a cough, with a typical "whoop", the effect of a vaccine would appear to be lower than if you only included people who also had those symptoms plus confirmation of the diagnosis by laboratory tests. Some of your cases of cough and whoop might not in fact be whooping cough, so the vaccine could not be expected to protect them. Only the cases with laboratory confirmation are true whooping cough. It pays to be strict in how you decide who is and who is not a case, as this gives you the best chance of finding out the true effect of the vaccine. Phase 3 trials nearly always require laboratory confirmation to be sure that a suspected case really is a case.

At the same time, you don't want to have a definition that is too restrictive. It has to be meaningful to the person you are trying to protect, so you might want to include less severe cases. The results for COVID-19 trials are often presented according to whether the vaccine prevents death, hospitalisation, milder cases and ability to stop transmission. Most Phase 3 trials will measure several outcomes (the technical term is *endpoints*). Efficacy is usually highest for hospitalisation and death, lower for mild disease and lowest for interruption of transmission. Knowing the efficacy of a vaccine against several different outcomes is very helpful in understanding what its impact in society would be.

Another challenge in a Phase 3 trial is finding all the cases. People with symptoms don't always go to their doctor, even if they are in a trial. Researchers go to great lengths to make it as easy as possible to find all the cases of a disease. They make sure the doctors in the area know about the study, and have the equipment to take any laboratory samples such as nose and throat swabs. Identifying all the cases is fairly straightforward in Europe and in the United States, but in Africa, where doctors are few and far between, it isn't so easy. In the Malawi rotavirus vaccine trial, the study was a regular radio feature. The study was explained in simple language, with the latest hit record playing in the background. Everyone in Malawi has a radio, so it was an effective way to reach a wide audience.

Recruitment to vaccine trials is challenging in both high- and low-income countries. I learned a few techniques over the years. It always pays to work with experienced centres who have done many trials and understand their local population. I avoided places where anti-vaccination sentiment was high. Communication, at the right level, is key. I became involved in developing a children's book that explained research to young schoolchildren in simple language with illustrations. In another trial, in teenagers, we used social media platforms designed by teenagers, to get messages across. Involvement of local community leaders helps build trust. One of the countries that was particularly good at recruiting young children to trials was Estonia. I spent several days there, talking to study nurses to work out how they did this. It boiled down to trust. The process of recruiting someone to a trial didn't happen at one visit. There were a series of community meetings to talk about the trial before recruitment even started. There was a strong culture of sharing experiences – positive and negative – between the nurses. They had created a community, over many years, where research was viewed positively.

The specific nature of vaccines also affects where the trials are conducted. Drug trials often take place in hospitals where patients with a particular condition are to be found. Vaccine trials take place where vaccines are given – in GP surgeries and community clinics. Each trial centre will only recruit a few volunteers, so a Phase 3 vaccine trial can involve thousands of centres, often in more than one country. One rotavirus vaccine trial in South America recruited babies from twelve countries. This creates all kinds of logistical problems. It takes time to train a centre on how to run a trial properly. Study monitors need to visit each centre regularly to check on the progress of the trial, ensure quality is being maintained and conduct more training if necessary. The study vaccines need to be kept properly refrigerated during transport and after arrival. A vaccine in a trial has a long journey, which starts at the manufacturing site. Study vaccines then need to be shipped to the countries where the trial is taking place. They have to clear customs, then delivered to a storage depot. From there, the vaccines are transported to all the study sites. They have to be kept at the right temperature, between two and eight degrees Centigrade, during this long journey. If the vaccine is exposed to excessive heat, it can't be used, which is a major setback; it can take months to manufacture a new batch of vaccine if something goes wrong. It is even more difficult in tropical countries where the vaccines have to withstand sweltering temperatures, and roads often flood in the rainy season. Clearing customs is another headache; planes carrying vaccines sometimes sit for hours on the tarmac in hot temperatures while the paperwork is sorted out. The requirement for some COVID-19 vaccines to be frozen at minus seventy degrees made the logistics of the clinical trials even more complicated.

It's a common belief that drug companies like to do research in developing countries because it's cheaper. My own experience was very different. Before we could start the rotavirus vaccine trial in Malawi, several health centres had to be completely renovated with reliable fridges, storage space and training facilities. Internet service had to be installed so trial information could be transmitted to our HQ in real time. This is particularly important for monitoring side effects. Land Rovers were bought that would be able to navigate the roads in the rainy season. Nurses and doctors had to be recruited and trained to conduct the trial to international standards. This capacity building is a recognised and accepted aspect of doing research in developing countries, provided it is appropriate and sustainable. Many of the recent COVID-19 trials were conducted in developing countries, not because they are cheaper, but because of the need to show the vaccine is effective where the need is greatest.

A Phase 3 trial is a huge investment. One trial of a vaccine for human papillomavirus (the virus that causes cancer of the cervix) that I was involved in recruited nearly 19,000 volunteers in fourteen countries, across 135 sites. More than 250,000 samples were tested. The trial ran for six and a half years. The budget was a €111 million. It is quite normal for the pharmaceutical industry to spend these amounts in Phase 3 trials.

In a Phase 3 trial there will usually be a team of people whose job it is to keep a close watch on the trial results as they come in. They are independent from both the company sponsoring the trial and the people who are actually conducting the trial. This is called an independent data monitoring committee (IDMC), sometimes also known as a data and safety monitoring board (DSMB). They meet periodically and review the data unblinded, in other words they get to see who has had the vaccine and who has had the control and what is the rate of side effects and disease in the two groups. They may recommend stopping the trial – either because the rate of side effects is too high, or because it becomes clear that the experimental vaccine is not going to work. If someone in the trial gets a severe reaction, they can pause the trial, while checks are carried to see if the reaction was due to the vaccine. They can also stop a trial early if it becomes apparent the vaccine is effective, so there is no need to recruit additional volunteers.

When all the volunteers have been recruited, received their vaccinations, had all their blood tests and the study monitors have completed their last visit, it is time for the moment of truth – analysing the results. The code that identifies volunteers as being in the vaccine group or the control group is broken, and the vaccine efficacy can be calculated.

Vaccine efficacy is easily misunderstood, as it is calculated based at a population level, not an individual level. The best way to think of the efficacy of a vaccine is that it is the percentage reduction in the risk of you catching a disease if you are vaccinated versus not being vaccinated. It's also worth noting that the larger the size of the Phase 3 trial, the more accurate will be the estimate of efficacy that is calculated. As well as giving the efficacy result, there will be a range, showing the upper and lower estimate. The efficacy estimate is the most likely correct result, but the range tells you it might be as low as x or as high as y. This range is called the confidence interval (sometimes also known as the credible interval).

The results of the COVID-19 Phase 3 trials have shown differences in efficacy, not just between vaccines, but also depending on the age group, the country where the trial was done, and whether you look at severe disease versus mild disease. This is to be expected. Efficacy tends to be lower in older people, as their immune systems age. Differences between countries can be due to a number of factors, for example whether there are different strains of the virus, or sometimes genetic differences. The efficacy of the COVID-19 vaccine made by Johnson & Johnson was 72% in the United States, 66% in South America, and 57% in South Africa. The lower protection in South America and South Africa was probably due to the presence of more infectious variants in those parts of the world; the emergence of variants has skewed the results of subsequent trials with other COVID-19 vaccines. In the Johnson & Johnson trial, there were differences in the level of protection depending on whether you looked at more severe disease. The overall efficacy was 66%, but for severe disease it rose to 85%. Higher efficacy against more severe disease is what you expect; you don't need complete protection to stop the worst effects of the virus whereas preventing all disease is a much higher bar.

Differences in efficacy between countries can sometimes also be due to genetic differences. When vaccines against *Haemophilus influenzae* type b (Hib), a serious bacterial infection of young children, were first introduced in the United States, they had a dramatic impact; however, the impact was much less for native Navajo, White Mountain Apache and Alaskan children. These differences were due to the specific genetic makeup of those populations.

A Phase 3 trial provides a great deal more information besides efficacy. The large number of vaccinations given in the trial provides much more accurate information about side effects. Less common side effects will be detected for the first time. More serious side effects will require further investigation, and possibly further trials, particularly if they are unexpected.

Phase 3 trials also provide very useful information about antibody responses to the vaccine. Because a Phase 3 trial is the first time that you can measure the efficacy of the vaccine, this information can be used to see what level of antibody is needed to protect. This is called the correlate of protection. Knowing the correlate of protection is very helpful. It means that in future trials, all you need to do to determine if a vaccine is effective, is to measure antibodies, which can be done in a much smaller number of people. The first COVID-19 vaccines were licensed on the basis of efficacy data in Phase 3 trials; second generation versions are being licensed on the basis of antibody results, which require fewer numbers. It isn't always possible to determine the correlate of protection, particularly for complex diseases that involve several components of the immune system to provide protection, such as malaria.

Antibody responses are measured for the new vaccine, but they are also measured for the other existing vaccines that are given at the same time. This is important, to check whether there is any interference between the new vaccine and the existing ones.

Finally, Phase 3 trials provide information that is critical to the future manufacturing process. Phase 1 and Phase 2 trials are done with vaccines that are produced in small batches, called clinical trial lots. In a Phase 3 trial, the vaccines are produced in large batches, which is what will happen when it goes into mass production – commercial lots. Being able to produce large numbers of doses, with consistency, is vital, as vaccines are needed for hundreds of millions of people. A Phase 3 vaccine trial will typically check the consistency of antibody responses between three large batches.

When the all the preclinical, and Phase 1, 2 and 3 studies have been finished, analysed and written up, the files can be sent to regulatory agencies around the world. This is a complicated process, as each country has its own legislation and requirements. In the United States, the agency that reviews files and decides whether a vaccine or drug can be authorised for use is the Food and Drug Administration, the FDA. In the European Union, there is one single agency, the European Medicines Agency, EMA, that grants authorisation on behalf of all the EU member states. File submissions run into several thousand pages. I worked on a vaccine against pneumococcal disease, which was in development for many years, with more than a dozen versions having been tried out. When we finally submitted the files to the European agency, they filled an entire lorry.

As well as submitting files to the agencies, companies and research institutions are increasingly obliged to publish their results – positive or negative. They are also expected to register their trials online. ClinicalTrials.gov is the biggest online register of trials. Transparency of research has increased greatly, but still needs to improve.

35

It used to be that Phase 3 was the end of the story for vaccine research. The results would be written up and sent to the regulatory agency who would license the vaccine. The vaccine could then be rolled out for general use.

It is very different nowadays. There is more and more emphasis on the research that happens after the vaccine is licensed – Phase 4. Vaccines given in clinical trials are done under perfect conditions but real life is very different. Vaccines are not always stored properly. People don't get vaccinated on time, and sometimes don't complete the course. However big a Phase 3 trial is, it still cannot detect the rarest side effects, or study the long-term effects of the vaccine. Blood clots following some COVID-19 vaccines occur at a rate of about 1 in 100,000. The Phase 3 trial only recruited around 30,000 people, so clots were only detected after millions of people had been vaccinated.

The aim of Phase 4 is to provide information on the safety and effectiveness of the vaccine in the conditions that they are actually used. In these real-life conditions, the effectiveness can be lower than was found in the Phase 3 trial, but it can also be higher. This is because when a vaccine is given to millions of people, it protects not only those who are vaccinated, but also reduces the risk of unvaccinated people catching the disease, so the overall impact is greater. This is being seen in countries that have rolled out COVID-19 vaccination with high uptake.

Phase 4 programmes also follow-up the on volunteers in the Phase 3 trial, usually for at least two years, and sometimes longer. This provides evidence of the long-term safety and effectiveness of the vaccine. The volunteers in the trial that first showed the effectiveness of measles vaccine in the UK were followed up for twenty-seven years. Not only were they still protected against measles, but many had given birth to babies who were also protected.

A Phase 4 programme is agreed during the licensing process and is a condition of the licence being granted. If the studies are not done, the licence can be revoked. Phase 4 vaccine programmes are often bigger than all the other phases put together. I worked on a shingles vaccine at GlaxoSmithKline. The file for the vaccine, which was first licensed in 2017, had clinical trial data on 30,000 volunteers. There are more than half a million participants in the Phase 4 studies, which will last to 2025.

So, what happened in the Malawi rotavirus vaccine trial? It turned out that efficacy of the rotavirus vaccine there was just below fifty percent. This was lower than in other countries – the trial also recruited babies in South Africa, where the efficacy was sixty-one percent. The lower efficacy was probably due to a number of factors. Children in developing countries suffer from many types of gut infections which can interfere with vaccines that are given by mouth. They are less well nourished, which lowers their ability to mount an immune response. Also, there may be more variants of the virus in Africa, some of which are not so easily prevented by vaccination. However, despite the lower efficacy in Malawi, the vaccine still had the potential to have a big impact, as the disease is so common there. For every 100 children vaccinated in Malawi during the trial, it was calculated that seven cases of severe diarrhoea due to rotavirus were prevented. In other words, you need to vaccinate about fourteen babies to prevent one case of severe illness. This is actually a very good result; in comparison it has been estimated that you need to vaccinate 256 adults in the UK to prevent one case of COVID-19. The results of the trials in Malawi and South Africa led to the World Health Organization recommending the use of the vaccine in the poorest countries of the world. Malawi introduced routine rotavirus vaccination for all babies in 2012; the number of infant deaths from diarrhoea there has since fallen by a third (many of the remaining deaths are caused by diseases other than rotavirus).

The development of the rotavirus vaccine took more than ten years. The trials for the first COVID-19 vaccines were completed in ten months. Surely this means that corners were cut?

There were several reasons why this accelerated timetable was possible. A lot of the preparatory work had already been done. The world has had two "near misses" of pandemics from other coronavirus infections: SARS (severe acute respiratory syndrome) in 2003 and MERS (Middle East respiratory syndrome) in 2012. Scientists had already worked on both and had done trials with experimental vaccines. Advances in technology, particularly in genetics, meant that it was possible to create an experimental vaccine against the new virus within days. The most important factor, however, was that companies, with massive investment from governments, were able to progress from one stage to the next much more rapidly. After a Phase 1 trial, a company would normally think long and hard about whether to move to Phase 2, where the costs start to rise rapidly. The cost of development was underwritten for several companies working on COVID-19 vaccines, with advance purchase orders should they succeed, and no loss if they failed. Freed of this financial risk, Phase 2 COVID-19 trials could start as soon as safety had been established in Phase 1. Phase 1 and 2 often overlapped, with Phase 2 starting as soon as it had been determined the vaccine was safe. Phase 3 trials followed rapidly; again, recruitment could start without having to worry about how likely they would be to succeed. Many more trial centres could be opened, enabling the required numbers to be recruited more rapidly. Regulatory agencies prioritised the review of the trial data, and when they did grant authorisation, it was for emergency use; these authorisations are being reviewed as more data arrive. The total number of volunteers recruited in these trials was no less than usual (in some cases rather more) and there was the same level of scrutiny. Trials were conducted to Good Clinical Practice, with ethics approval, regulatory inspections and oversight by independent data monitoring committees. In short, the same amount of research was done as in a conventional development, but in less time. Also, the trials are not over; the participants will be followed up for years, providing further information on the many unknowns, such as how long protection lasts, the effectiveness against mutant strains, and whether the vaccine prevents transmission as well as disease. The development of COVID-19 vaccines has been a triumph for science. Trials have been conducted all over the world, in the most challenging circumstances, without compromising quality or patient safety. Vaccine research has come a long way since Jenner and Pasteur's primitive experiments. Good science prevails (even if you have to occasionally beware of the crocodiles).

The Space Shuttle

My medical training lasted six years. In all that time we had one lecture on vaccination. I spent another five years training in public health, where I learned quite a lot about vaccination, and how vaccination services are organised. I then worked for fifteen years at the UK's national public health centre, where I specialised in vaccines. I studied the epidemiology of diseases like measles, whooping cough and meningitis, did clinical trials of several vaccines, wrote scientific papers and sat on all kinds of expert committees. I was the co-editor of *Immunisation against Infectious Disease*, the handbook (nowadays online) that describes vaccination policy in the UK. In short, I became a vaccine nerd. Surely, I knew everything about vaccines that mattered? Actually, no. Until I visited a vaccine manufacturing site, I was pretty clueless about how they were actually made. I knew the general principles, but if asked to describe the manufacturing process in detail, I would have struggled. Most doctors and nurses who give vaccines on a daily basis have only a rudimentary knowledge about what they contain and how they are made.

The reality is that vaccine manufacturing is an extraordinarily complex process. After my job at the UK Public Health Institute, I moved to Belgium, to work at the headquarters of GlaxoSmithKline's vaccine business. The manufacturing site there is humongous. Covering an area the size of seventy football pitches, it employs 7,000 highly skilled workers who produce 2 million vaccine doses a day. One of the first things I did when I arrived was to take a tour of the facilities. The scale and complexity bowled me over. The head of manufacturing, John McGrath, a genial Irishman, described it beautifully: he said that making Anadin was like designing a really nice racing bike, an antibody was like manufacturing a Boeing 787, but a modern vaccine was like building the Space Shuttle.

Vaccines are very different from drugs. They are made from biological materials, including living organisms such as viruses. This brings uncertainty to the manufacturing process. The flu virus that grows like a weed one year may not be so co-operative the following year. Like wine, there are good years and bad years, depending on the yield. There isn't an endless supply of the source materials. Many are highly specialised products, with a limited number of suppliers. The vaccine recipe book contains some familiar ingredients like gelatin, glycine, formaldehyde and enzymes. It also has some rather fancier components. One of these are the cells that are needed for the viruses to grow on, without risk of contamination (bacterial vaccines, in contrast, are grown on nutrient broth, which is widely available). The cells used for viral culture are highly treasured, and cannot easily be replaced or substituted. Some of these cells have been in continuous use since the 1960s, for example MRC-5 (named after the UK Medical Research Council, that originally created the cell line, at their fifth attempt). There has been a lot of ethical debate about the use of cells in vaccine production, particularly since some originate from cells derived from an aborted fetus. The cells used in vaccine production are descended from the original cell but do not contain any original ingredients. There are now several different types of cells used for growing viruses. Not all viruses are grown on cells. Some, for example influenza, are grown in chick eggs. These are not the sort of eggs that you buy in a supermarket. They come

DOI: 10.1201/9781003303879-8

39

from highly controlled flocks, and there is a limited supply. Culturing a flu virus in eggs is rather inefficient, with each vaccine dose needing one egg. As there are four different strains of virus in flu vaccine, you need four eggs to make one vaccine. There just aren't that many chickens.

The most specialised ingredient of all is the seed lot, which is the batch of virus or bacterium that is the starting point for manufacture. A seed lot is made from a master seed bank which in turn is derived from the original strain that was first used to make the vaccine, many years earlier. For example, most rubella (German measles) vaccines today are made from a strain of the virus called RA 27/3, which has been in use for fifty years. These strains can be relied upon to produce vaccines in large quantities. For any one vaccine there are usually only a handful of virus strains that are available for production. The advent of genetic vaccines has simplified the manufacturing process, although most vaccines in use today still rely on traditional methods.

Vaccines and drugs are both made in spotlessly clean environments, to avoid contamination. The sterile requirements for vaccines, however, are in a different league. Many vaccines are made from living viruses or bacteria, which have to be kept in the highest possible level of containment so they cannot escape. The manufacturing environment must be completely sterile. Air supplies are changed continually, and tested to make sure they are free from bacteria or other contaminants. Everything that is possible to clean, is cleaned, following rigid protocols. Environmental swabs are continuously taken from floors, ceilings and equipment to look for any sign of contamination with bacteria. Factory workers wear disposable masks and gowns. The changing rooms in a vaccine site look more like an operating theatre than a factory. To avoid cross-contamination, each different vaccine is usually made separately, in its own building, with dedicated equipment and employees.

Every step of the process is documented and carried out to standard operating procedures (SOPs). The number of SOPs in a large vaccine manufacturing site runs into the thousands. There are quality control tests at every stage, with strict defined standards to be met. One of the vaccines which protects against pneumococcal disease in babies has to pass over 500 quality control tests during its manufacture. More people work on quality control in a vaccine manufacturing site than work on the actual production.

Vaccine manufacturing is highly regulated. A manufacturer has to satisfy the demands of the country where the site is located, but also the countries where the vaccines will eventually be used. Regulatory authorities frequently send inspectors to vaccines sites. These inspectors, who can arrive unannounced, are very, very fastidious. They have checklists that run into hundreds of pages. They are there to find mistakes, and when they spot one, they dig, and keep digging. A team of inspectors may spend several days at a site, poring over records, taking samples and interviewing employees. At the end of the inspection, they give their assessment. At best, this will be a list of things that need to be fixed, such as better documentation of cleaning, which will be checked the next time they come. If there are more serious shortcomings, they can halt production altogether. In 2004, one flu vaccine manufacturer had their licence suspended because of concerns about possible contamination of product. They were scheduled to produce nearly 50 million doses of vaccine for the United States, so overnight, the flu vaccine supply for the country was cut in half.

Because of the less predictable nature of viruses and bacteria, any change in the manufacturing process creates uncertainty about the impact on the final product. Changes in the process can happen for many reasons – new equipment, changes in raw materials, a new facility, or changes in the regulations. New clinical trials may be needed to check that change has not affected the safety or effectiveness of the vaccine. Conducting a trial on a vaccine which is already licensed, for the sole purpose of checking the impact of a process change, is difficult, as there is little incentive for people to participate. Imagine being invited to join a trial in which you will receive a vaccine that you can get anyway from your doctor without having to go through all the blood tests, when the purpose of the trial is to test whether a change in the way the vaccine is made has affected its safety or effectiveness. Manufacturers try to avoid having to do these trials whenever possible, and look for other ways to validate the process change.

The extraordinary complexity of vaccine manufacturing means that there are relatively few companies who are able to produce consistently high-quality vaccines in large enough quantities. The investment in time and people is daunting. To build and commission a new factory from scratch takes five to seven years, at a cost which can exceed €1 billion. There are only a handful of companies who make vaccines on a global scale, although the COVID-19 pandemic is changing this. Before COVID-19, more than ninety percent of all the vaccines in Europe and the United States were made by one of just four companies: Merck, Pfizer, GlaxoSmithKline and Sanofi Pasteur. Now, there is a slew of new kids on the block: Moderna, Novavax, Johnson & Johnson, AstraZeneca and others. Outside of Europe and the United States, a few countries are also able to produce vaccines at scale: Japan, China, India, Brazil and Russia have thriving vaccine industries which are mainly focused on their domestic markets. COVID-19 is also changing this; the Russian Sputnik V vaccine is licensed in many countries outside Russia, including in Europe (in February 2021 Hungary became the first ever country in Europe to use a Russian-made vaccine). Two Chinese-made COVID-19 vaccines have been approved by the World Health Organization for distribution through the COVAX scheme that aims to ensure equitable distribution of COVID-19 vaccines. They are being rolled out in Asia, Africa, South America and Europe. Technology transfers are enabling vaccines to be manufactured where they are needed; AstraZeneca's vaccine is now being made by the State Serum Institute of India, for its massive population. Vaccine manufacturing is still highly complex but thanks to international co-operation it is possible on a much bigger, more rapid scale. The Space Shuttle is now more like the International Space Station, a multinational collaborative effort. Expansion and diversification of the vaccine industry is a good thing. Reliance on a handful of suppliers is a headache for governments who need to organise vaccination programmes. A sudden surge in demand – for example during an epidemic, or a migrant crisis, places a big strain on manufacturing capacity. A major quality issue with one manufacturer's vaccine will mean others have to step in to meet the demand. This means that temporary interruptions in supply are inevitable, particularly for new vaccines, as teething troubles are ironed out. It came as no surprise all three of the companies that first produced COVID-19 vaccines had supply issues within weeks of being approved.

I now invite you to join me in building the Space Shuttle. The first step is assembling all the raw materials. This takes a bit of time as they are not widely available. A drug usually has just one chemical compound, plus a few materials to formulate it into a pill, syrup or injection. A vaccine uses up to twenty different types of ingredients. The most important is the virus or bacterium that will be used to make the active ingredient. Many vaccines contain more than one strain of the active ingredient. One of the vaccines for pneumococcal infection contains twenty strains (called serotypes) of the bacterium *Streptococcus pneumoniae*, each one of which will eventually be joined to a protein during manufacture in a process called conjugation. The viruses and bacteria need to be grown on something, so cells and culture media are needed.

An adjuvant is an important ingredient for some vaccines. These performance-enhancing substances are very useful from a manufacturing perspective. With an improved immune response, it is possible to lower the amount of the active component in the vaccine and make more doses. This can be critical when manufacturing needs to be ramped up quickly, for example in a response to a flu pandemic. The science of adjuvants has mushroomed in recent years. Many naturally derived products have been found to enhance the immune response to vaccines. Squalene is an oil found in many plants and animals, especially sharks. The oil that lubricates human skin and hair contains squalene. It is used as an adjuvant for some flu vaccines. Another adjuvant, monophosphoryl liquid (MPL) is isolated from the surface of a type of salmonella bacteria. The ingredients of these modern bespoke adjuvants are not so easy to come by. For example, one adjuvant is derived from a plant extract from a soap bark tree, *Quillaja saponaria*, which grows only in central Chile, in protected plantations.

Preservatives are often added to keep the vaccine free from contamination by bacteria. Stabilisers are also needed; these do exactly what they say, keeping the vaccine stable under different conditions of heat, freezing and drying. To make life even more complicated, some vaccines are combinations, protecting against several diseases. Many vaccines given to babies are combinations; these contain up to thirty ingredients counting all the viruses, bacteria, adjuvant, stabilisers and preservative.

As many of these ingredients are biological products, they cannot be stored indefinitely, so have to be freshly prepared. They also have to be checked before use to ensure they meet all the quality specifications. It takes on average two weeks to assemble all the necessary ingredients for a vaccine.

Now comes the really tricky part: the virus or bacterium has to be cultured and harvested. Vaccines are manufactured in bioreactors, gleaming cylinders that wouldn't look out of place in a modern distillery. They hold up to 5,000 litres, producing batches which contain hundreds of thousands of doses, and can be as many as 2 million doses. To guarantee this level of output requires a high yield from the culture. The difficulty in making enough bulk product is one of the biggest rate-limiting factors in vaccine manufacture. The arrival of gene-based vaccines has helped overcome this bottleneck. The first genetically engineered vaccine was hepatitis B. The genetic material of the virus is inserted into a "host" organism (in this case, baker's yeast) which then instructs the organism to produce the virus – or at least the part that is needed for immunity – in massive quantities. This technique has revolutionised vaccine manufacture. Stockouts of hepatitis B vaccine are rare, simply because it is relatively easy to produce in large amounts. The gene-based methods now being used for some COVID-19 vaccines have made manufacturing even easier. The genetic material of the harmful part of the virus, the spike protein, is created in the laboratory, which takes just a few days. This is used to make either a DNA-based vaccine, inserting the genetic material into a harmless carrier virus, or an RNA-based vaccine, in which the genetic material goes straight into a vaccine after being wrapped in a protective coat. The great advantage of these modern gene-based vaccines is that they are easier and quicker to make than conventional ones. The laborious process of growing the virus, which takes several weeks, with an uncertain outcome, is no longer needed. Once you know the genetic structure of the virus, a vaccine can be made in days. When new variants come along, the vaccine can be quickly adjusted. A simplified manufacturing process allows more much more rapid scale up of production. The scale of manufacturing of COVID-19 vaccines is unprecedented and would almost certainly not have been possible with conventional manufacturing methods.

Despite the relative ease of making gene-based vaccines, most vaccines in use today are still made by the traditional method of growing the virus or bacterium over several weeks. These methods are tried and tested, and produce high-quality vaccines at scale. Switching production of an existing vaccine to a gene-based method would be a huge effort, with all the stages of trials having to be repeated. This will happen eventually, particularly where a gene-based vaccine can give better protection than a conventional one, but conventional vaccines are likely to be here for many years to come.

A critical aspect of vaccine manufacture is to produce a vaccine that is capable of stimulating the immune system, but without producing any symptoms of the disease. Traditionally, this is done by either inactivation (killing the virus or bacterium) or attenuation (weakening it to make it harmless). The oldest method is inactivation, using a chemical such as formalin. Formalin is a solution of formaldehyde with a characteristic strong, irritating smell. It is widely used for long-term storage of animal and organ specimens; if you have an aquarium, you probably used it to kill the parasites that live in fish. Formalin inactivation is a very reliable method still used today for many vaccines. Some of the most widely used vaccines in the world still use this method, such as polio and influenza. The other most common method is attenuation, where the virus or bacterium is grown repeatedly in cell cultures, which has the effect of weakening them. The attenuated organisms are still able to replicate, but they have lost their ability to cause disease. Measles, mumps, rubella and yellow fever are all examples of live attenuated vaccines.

The advent of modern manufacturing techniques – subunit and gene-based vaccines – has solved the problem of making the virus or bacterium harmless. These vaccines are not capable of multiplying; they also contain less active ingredient so have fewer side effects.

The final step in bulk manufacture is to clean the vaccine, to remove any impurities. During production, various by-products can end up in the vaccine; bits of cell walls, fragments of DNA and toxins. The vaccine is purified with a variety of chemical and physical methods such as filtration (which catches larger bits of unwanted material), centrifugation (spinning it rapidly) and chromatography, a technique used to separate chemicals travelling at different speeds through a column. Each vaccine is unique and has its own purification system.

The length of time for bulk manufacture varies depending on the vaccine, but it can take up to twelve months. Quality tests are carried out at every step – failure in a quality test can mean discarding the batch and starting all over again.

The next step is to assemble all the various ingredients together – the active viral or bacterial antigens, stabilisers, buffers, adjuvants and preservatives. This step is called formulation, it takes about a week, and marks the end of what is known as primary production. As well as the manufacturer's own quality control tests, at this stage the product will usually be tested by the regulatory agency in the country where it has been made.

All that remains is to fill, label and transport the vaccines. This is secondary production and is sometimes done at a different site from primary production. Sounds relatively straightforward, surely? No.

Vaccines are used all over the world, and every country has its own requirements. The vaccine might be put into a vial, or a pre-filled syringe. Vials can be single or multi-dose. The vaccine has to remain stable during its shelf life, which is typically two to three years. This can either be done by adding a chemical, or by a process called lyophilisation. In the process of lyophilisation, the vaccine is transformed into a powder by freeze-drying, which is much easier to keep preserved. A lyophilised vaccine is dissolved in a liquid, known as a diluent, at the time of the injection. The diluent is usually water or saline.

When the vaccine – liquid or lyophilised – has been bottled in vials, it needs to be labelled. The information on the label has to be in the local language, and each country has its own regulations about how the labelling is done, what product information needs to be included, and the instructions for whoever will give the vaccine – prescribing information. The requirements of countries change continuously and sometimes without warning. Keeping on top of the regulations of over a hundred countries is no mean feat. Vaccine companies have teams of people whose job it is to do this.

It takes several months to produce a final product that is ready to be shipped around the world; however before this can happen, there is another critical step – batch release. The manufacturer carries out a final series of quality checks to make sure the vaccine has been produced correctly. The local regulatory agency in the country of manufacture also carries out its own independent tests, and there will be further independent testing by the regulatory agencies of the countries to where the vaccine will be shipped. Some countries don't have the capacity to conduct their own testing. In this case, it will be carried out by an independent accredited agency, such as the UK National Institute for Biological Standards and Control in Potters Bar, just north of London. No vaccine can be shipped without passing this process of batch release.

The quality tests for vaccine batch release are complex and can take several weeks. One failed test can be enough to write off an entire batch, or at the very least delay its shipment. Only then can the vaccine start its journey to clinics, pharmacies and surgeries.

Shipment of vaccines is completely different from drugs for one reason. Most vaccines have to be kept between two and eight degrees Centigrade; a few have to be transported frozen (for example, some COVID-19 vaccines, but also one of the shingles vaccines). They are biological products and any temperature deviations, either below or above the storage limits, mean the vaccine may no longer be active. Vaccines are highly intrepid travellers. A vaccine can leave a manufacturing site in Europe in a lorry, go to the airport and take a plane to the other side of the world. Then it takes another lorry to a warehouse, joining other travelling companions. From there it has to get to the clinics. This might mean a Land Rover across the sweltering African savannah, a rickety boat ride up the Mekong Delta, or a hair-raising plane landing at 3,000 metres in Nepal. The process of preserving vaccines at the right temperature during their travels is called the cold chain, and has become a scientific discipline in its own right. Vaccines are transported in specially designed cold boxes, and every single shipment has a monitor that records any deviations in temperature during the journey. These monitors track the temperature record of the vaccine on its entire journey from the factory to the fridge in the clinic where it is used. If the vaccine is exposed to a temperature outside the recommended range, this is recorded on the monitor. If the deviation means the vaccine can no longer be used, the monitor changes colour. Ewan McGregor, the swashbuckling hero of *Star Wars*, made a documentary a few years ago about the cold chain, following the journey of vaccines to some of the most inaccessible communities on the planet. By coincidence I am from the same small Scottish town as Ewan; his dad taught me at school! The cold chain does not stop when a vaccine reaches its final destination. It has to be kept at the right temperature until it is used. Some vaccines are more resistant to temperature changes than others, but many won't survive for more than a day at room temperature. If the cleaner pulls out the plug of a vaccine fridge by mistake on Saturday morning, the clinic on Monday will have to be cancelled.

The whole process – bulk manufacture, formulation, filling and labelling, batch release and shipping – takes on average eighteen months, but can be up to three years. Every step of the journey is quality tested. There is no medicine, or any other consumable product that comes even close to the complexity of end-to-end vaccine manufacture. The next time you go for your annual flu injection or take your baby for their MMR vaccination, you have travelled on the Space Shuttle.

9

It's Not the Vicar's Fault!

Nothing in medicine has caused more controversy than the safety of vaccines. Soon after people started using Jenner's smallpox vaccine, cartoonists drew pictures of people turning into cows, sprouting horns and tails. No medical intervention is surrounded by more myths than vaccination. Ignorance, fear and misinformation have fuelled anti-vaccination sentiment. In the 1970s, vaccination rates in the UK plummeted to an all-time low because of fears of the safety of whooping cough vaccine, subsequently found to be greatly exaggerated. Later, an alleged link between measles/mumps/rubella (MMR) vaccine and autism would create a media frenzy that dominated newspaper headlines in the UK for years. This link was shown to be completely unfounded, however, the story ran and ran. I had a very personal involvement with the whole saga. I met Andrew Wakefield in 1992, when I was working at the UK National Public Health Institute. It was clear that he had an unshakeable belief in his theory, and would go to the ends of the earth to try and prove it. Although he was eventually completely discredited and banned from medical practice, this did not stop the media from running the story. I saw public confidence in MMR vaccine evaporate, and measles outbreaks return with a vengeance. I talked a lot to the media during this time. The health correspondent of one UK tabloid privately acknowledged that they appreciated that MMR vaccine did not cause autism; however, as their job is to write newsworthy copy, they weren't going to stop covering the story. They were very dark times. The "Wakefield effect" spread into Europe and later to the United States, where he now lives. MMR vaccination rates did not recover for more than twenty years. If you want to read the whole story, I recommend Brian Deer's book, *The Doctor Who Fooled the World*.

Vaccine safety is newsworthy. Vaccines are given to healthy people, often babies, in the millions. They are injected. They contain chemicals. The perfect storm. In this chapter, I'm going to talk about side effects that are actually caused by vaccines, how they are monitored, and also explain how statistics on the safety of vaccines can be very misleading (and yes, why it's not the vicar's fault).

Minor side effects (also called adverse events) are quite common. The most common are local reactions that occur under the skin at the site where the vaccine is injected. When you inject a vaccine into a muscle, it triggers a local inflammation. Within minutes, immune cells gather at the injection site, like soldiers responding to a foreign invasion. These soldiers trigger off a chain of events, stimulating your body to produce various chemicals – cytokines, chemokines, amines, bradykinin to name just a few. Your body is starting to develop an immune response. The result is often some swelling, which can be red and painful. This usually appears a day or two after the injection and nearly always disappears completely within a few days. The exception is the vaccine against tuberculosis, which creates a vigorous response at the injection site, often leaving a permanent scar. I'm sure many of you will remember receiving this vaccine and seeing a blister develop over the next few weeks, eventually forming a scab, which gradually heals.

DOI: 10.1201/9781003303879-9

As well as the local reaction, the immune cells and chemicals spill into your bloodstream, reaching other parts of the body, including your brain. This sets off other events that can cause more general symptoms. This is called a systemic reaction and the most common symptom is a fever. Other systemic reactions are similar to those that often occur when you have an infection – aching muscles, headache, no appetite, generally feeling under the weather. The difference with a vaccine is that the active ingredient has been weakened or killed, so the systemic reaction you experience with a vaccine is much less than with the real thing. Systemic reactions, like local ones, usually disappear in a couple of days.

I described the different types of vaccine, and adjuvants, in Chapter 4. Vaccines which contain the largest amounts of active ingredient will provoke the most ferocious response from the defending army and cause the most reactions. The first whooping cough vaccines, in the 1950s, were made from the entire bacterium, known as a whole cell vaccine. None of the components of the bacterium were removed in the manufacturing process. Whole cell whooping cough vaccines contained around 3,000 different components, however, only a handful of these were really needed to stimulate an immune response. These vaccines were very effective, but local and systemic reactions were common. Starting in the 1990s, whooping cough vaccines were made by selecting just the bits that are needed to provoke an immune response, the antigens. These "subunit" vaccines have just three to five antigens and cause fewer reactions. This means they can be safely combined with other vaccines in the same syringe, reducing the number of injections. One of the most common combinations given to babies protects against six diseases, however, even this multi-purpose vaccine contains only ten antigens, a fraction of the number in the early whooping cough vaccines.

Some vaccines also contain an adjuvant, to improve the immune response. There is a downside to this; an adjuvant tends to increase the side effects of the vaccine. For example, one of the vaccines for shingles contains an adjuvant. After two doses of the vaccine roughly two-thirds of people will have experienced a sore arm, and a third will have had muscle aches or fatigue. These symptoms resolve within a day or two.

A major source of anxiety about vaccine safety is that they contain chemicals that are perceived to be harmful. The reality is that these chemicals are either not present at all, or if they are present, they are in lower amounts than we are exposed to on a daily basis through food, water and other natural sources. The one that has attracted the most attention is thiomersal. Thiomersal is a derivative of mercury, and for many years was used in the process of manufacturing vaccines as a preservative. Several vaccines contained traces of thiomersal in the end product. Although this was well below the level that is harmful, it has been removed from all vaccines given to children for the last twenty years. Traces of thiomersal are still present in a few vaccines given to adults, at levels well below those found in nature.

Because some vaccines are made with a tame version of the real thing, they can also cause a mild version of the disease. This only happens with live attenuated vaccines, which replicate inside your body to provoke an immune response. Measles vaccine, for example, can cause "mini measles" with a rash and fever which appears between five and twelve days after vaccination, the same incubation period as the natural infection. Rubella (better known as German measles) is also a live vaccine, and can similarly cause a mild version of the disease, including the rash, as well as joint pain, and occasionally a drop in platelets, the blood cells that are responsible for clotting. The vaccine version of the disease is however always much less severe than the real thing.

More serious reactions do occur, but fortunately are rare. Occasionally there is a very severe allergic response, called anaphylaxis, with hives, swelling of the lips and tongue, and breathing difficulty. Anaphylaxis is serious, but it can be treated with adrenaline. Vaccination clinics keep a stock of adrenaline in case this happens. In the UK, before COVID-19 vaccination began, there were on average eighteen cases a year of anaphylaxis following vaccination. This may sound a lot, but to put it in context, more than 16 million doses of vaccine were given every year. In comparison, forty-nine people are struck by lightning every year in the UK. With the mass roll out of COVID-19 vaccines, there have inevitably been more reports of anaphylaxis; however, it is still an extremely rare event. Deaths from vaccine-related anaphylaxis are virtually non-existent.

Another serious, but rare, immune-related side effect is Guillain–Barré syndrome (GBS). In GBS, the immune system turns on itself, damaging nerve cells, causing weakness and sometimes paralysis. This usually occurs in adults above fifty years of age. Most people recover completely but some are left with long-term disability. The exact cause of GBS isn't known, although it often occurs after a viral or bacterial infection. There has been a huge amount of research into whether vaccines can cause GBS. The only one where there may be a genuine link is the flu vaccine; GBS occurs about in about one per million people who get vaccinated. It's worth pointing out that this is lower than the risk of contracting GBS due to flu; you're almost twenty times more likely to get GBS if you catch flu versus getting the vaccine.

Despite the massive roll out of COVID-19 vaccines (over 11 billion doses at the time of writing), serious side effects are rare. Blood clots with low platelets have been reported after the AstraZeneca and Johnson & Johnson vaccines and heart inflammation following the Pfizer and Moderna vaccines.

The bottom line is that the more serious vaccine side effects are very rare, and people nearly always recover completely. These effects have to be weighed against the risks from catching the diseases. In this respect, vaccination is the victim of its own success. Vaccines have been so successful at eliminating diseases that the focus has turned to the side effects. Unfortunately, when people stop vaccinating, the diseases come back with a vengeance. Look at what's happened to measles: the disease was close to elimination until people stopped vaccinating because of the fear of autism linked to MMR vaccine. Vaccination rates are now recovering, but the damage has been done. There are outbreaks of measles all over Europe. The disease is at its highest level this century, with more than 100,000 cases in 2019 alone, and almost 100 deaths over the past four years. Contrast this with polio. High vaccination rates have been maintained and the disease is close to eradication.

Because vaccines are given to healthy people, it's tempting to conclude that anything that happens afterwards must be due to the vaccine. This is logical for the common side effects like swollen arms and fever. But anything else may simply have occurred by chance. People become ill all the time, so it's inevitable that sometimes their symptoms will start soon after vaccination. Autism is usually diagnosed at around eighteen months of age. This is exactly the age at which the MMR vaccine is given. It is, however, incorrect to conclude the vaccine is the culprit. Unvaccinated babies also develop autism, and autism was around long before MMR vaccine was invented. A more relevant statistic is whether autism is more common in children who have been vaccinated compared to those who have not. When you do this analysis, the link disappears. The recommended vaccination schedule in the UK requires a child to be vaccinated at six different visits by their fifth birthday. Any parent will tell you that illnesses are common in young children. It is inevitable that by coincidence, some symptoms will start soon after vaccination. That doesn't mean it's the fault of the vaccine. I will never forget attending a lecture by Euan Ross, who was the professor of paediatrics at the Royal Free Hospital in London. I had just started my public health training, and the lecture was at the Royal College of Physicians, a rather austere 1960s building in a quiet cul-de-sac off Regent's Park. Euan is a benign, bespectacled figure, with a twinkle in his eye and a wicked sense of humour. He was talking about convulsions following whooping cough vaccination. This was a hot topic at the time, with many parents deciding against the vaccine because they thought it caused fits. He explained that fits are actually a common event in babies. The risk of a three- to six-month-old baby having a fit within any five-day period is calculated to be 1 in 15,000. Babies are usually christened between three and six months of age, therefore 1 in 15,000 babies will have a fit within five days of the happy event. "It's not the vicar's fault!" he proclaimed triumphantly, donning his trademark imp-ish grin.

In 1965, an English statistician, Sir Austin Bradford Hill, laid out a set of principles to deter-mine whether a disease that occurs after an intervention is caused by it. In other words, if Y (for example blood clots) happens after X (COVID-19 vaccination) does X cause Y? The Bradford Hill criteria are still the basis for determining causality and have been widely used to investigate links between vaccines and reported side effects. They criteria has been adopted by the World Health Organization and many other public health agencies. Bradford Hill proposed nine crite-ria. The more that are met, the more likely there is a genuine cause and effect. Some of the criteria are "must haves" – failure to meet the criterion rules out the possibility of a causal link.

Bradford Hill criteria are: strength of association, consistency, specificity, temporality, bio-logical gradient, plausibility, coherence, experiment and analogy. That's rather a mouthful, but as these criteria are still widely used today it's worth looking at them in more detail.

- *Strength of association*. How much more frequently does the side effect occur after being vaccinated compared to not being vaccinated? If studies show that you are 100 times more likely to develop a reaction if you get a vaccine compared to not getting the vaccine, that's much more convincing than if you are just twice as likely to get the reaction after the vaccine.
- *Consistency (also called reproducibility)*. If a condition following vaccination has been found in many studies, in different countries and age groups, then a link is more plausible than if it is a one-off finding. The allegation that MMR vaccine caused autism is a great example of not meeting this criterion. It was originally made by one researcher, Andrew Wakefield. Since then, many researchers have tried to reproduce his alleged results. Not one has succeeded.
- *Specificity*. Is it just one condition that occurs after the vaccine or is it a number of similar conditions? And does it only occur after one type of vaccine or after many different types? The more specific the condition, and the vaccine, the more plausible the link. One in a million people will develop paralysis after receiving the live oral polio vaccine. This is a specific condition with classic symptoms. It only occurs after live polio vaccine, not any other vaccine (including the killed polio vaccine). The link has been clearly established (it meets the other criteria as well).
- *Temporality*. The condition must have started after the vaccination, not before it. This might seem obvious, but it can be hard to pin down an exact date for when a condition started, particularly for long-term conditions, which evolve slowly. There have been many claims that vaccines cause autoimmune disorders. These are illnesses in which you are attacked by your own immune system. Psoriasis, multiple sclerosis and inflammatory bowel disease are examples of autoimmune disorders. When you look into the date on which the very first symptoms began, they often start before the vaccine, so the association no longer holds water. Temporality is a must-have criterion.
- *Biological gradient* (also known as dose–response). If the side effect increases in severity or frequency with a higher dose of vaccine or with repeat exposure, then this makes it more likely the association is real. In practice, most vaccines are given at a standard dose, with a fixed number of doses, so it isn't possible to make meaningful comparisons between different levels of exposure.

- *Plausibility*. Is there a reasonable scientific explanation for how the vaccine could have caused the condition? Paralysis following oral polio vaccine is readily explained by the fact that the virus in the vaccine is known to occasionally change back to a more virulent form and that the real disease causes a type of paralysis which is identical to the one that occurs after the vaccine. On the other hand, there is no plausible explanation as to how MMR vaccine could cause autism.
- *Coherence*. This is similar to plausibility. There may be scientific data – laboratory experiments, epidemiology studies, case histories – which can contribute to the understanding of a newly observed link. The more you can use these data to weave a coherent picture of what might be happening, the more likely it is to be real.
- *Experiment*. If you can demonstrate the link, by replicating the exposure and the outcome in an experimental situation, it becomes more convincing. This criterion is rarely used nowadays as it usually involves exposing animals in experiments which are not acceptable by today's standards.
- *Analogy*. Are there other examples of a link that are already known? If a causal link has already been established between one vaccine and a condition, and you then see the same condition with a similar type of vaccine, it's more likely to be real. The fact that blood clots have appeared with two COVID-19 vaccines that use the same technology make it more probable that there is a causal association.

Bradford Hill criteria are a great framework for rational thinking as it's very easy to let your own biases distort the facts.

The assessment of vaccine safety starts with clinical trials. At every stage, trials actively follow-up study volunteers to look for side effects, and as described in Chapter 7, there are also studies set up to check for side effects after the vaccine is approved. These studies are not the end of vaccine safety assessment however, far from it. The safety of a vaccine is monitored continuously, for as long as it is on the market. Every country has a reporting system for vaccine side effects. Some systems are more sophisticated than others. In Europe, doctors are required to report all suspected vaccine side effects, even if the side effect is already recognised. There are additional reporting requirements for new vaccines, which have a "black triangle" – an inverted triangle symbol that appears on the leaflets that come with the vaccine and on any advertisements. Manufacturers also have legal reporting obligations, as they also get to hear about side effects. They have to submit regular summaries of these reports – Periodic Safety Update Reports – to the European regulatory agency. These include reports on side effects that occur anywhere in the world, not just in Europe. The UK has its own agency that has the same function, the Medicines and Healthcare Regulatory Agency (MHRA), as does the USA (which has three complementary vaccine safety monitoring schemes).

These reporting schemes provide very useful information, but can be difficult to interpret. Reporting is biased towards more serious side effects, particularly if they occur soon after vaccination. There is under-reporting: busy doctors may not report something, especially if it is mild or they are not sure it was caused by the vaccine. Safety monitoring schemes are most useful for newly introduced vaccines; vaccinators are more wary of something they are less familiar with, so are more likely to report a side effect. Despite their limitations, these reporting systems are good for signal detection – identifying something new or unexpected which can then be further investigated. Electronic records are making a big difference in vaccine safety monitoring, as vaccination data become increasingly linked to hospital records and general practitioner consultations. Social media are now being used as a way of picking up information on vaccine side effects, and soon it will be possible to use personal health monitoring devices to detect signals.

The follow-up of vaccine side effects has also become more sophisticated by the development of an international set of standards to describe side effects. The Brighton Collaboration is a network of scientists who have established agreed-upon definitions for each side effect. The collaboration started after a scientific meeting in Brighton, where Bob Chen, an epidemiologist from the US Centers for Disease Control and Prevention (CDC), gave a presentation on the need to standardise the methods for collecting vaccine safety information. I got to know Bob many years earlier when I spent six months at the CDC in Atlanta. He is a cheerful, unassuming character, passionate about vaccine safety, who has brought scientific rigour to the subject, enhancing the quality and consistency of data.

When a new side effect is picked up, a dedicated study is often needed to tease out what is actually happening. By definition these will be rare events, too infrequent to have been detected during the clinical trials. Studies into vaccine safety are complex, and often prone to bias, particularly if there has been a lot of publicity about the side effect. In 2009, a vaccine was made against a new strain of influenza, H1N1. The vaccine was only used for a short time, in a few countries, as the epidemic turned out to be less serious than expected. There were soon reports of narcolepsy (sleeping sickness) following vaccination, especially from Finland where the vaccine had been extensively used. This quickly became big news with daily newspaper headlines. Many studies were carried out to determine whether the vaccine caused the illness. These have come up with different results and conclusions; however, they all acknowledge the bias that the publicity caused.

Our knowledge about vaccine safety has advanced enormously in recent years. However, our understanding is mostly at the population level. At the individual level it can be very hard to determine whether an event that happened after the vaccination was caused by it, or just a chance coincidence. When someone develops a serious illness, we want an explanation, even if it is not rational. A recent vaccination is a likely scapegoat. Someone who develops an illness shortly after being vaccinated will quite reasonably assume it was caused by the vaccine, whatever the data at the population level might say. There is no laboratory test that can say for sure whether or not an illness was caused by a vaccine in an individual.

The vast majority of vaccinations are given with no side effects, or minor, short-lived ones. More serious side effects are rare, but they do occur. It boils down to a balance of benefit versus risk; to what extent can we tolerate side effects to prevent illnesses which can be life threatening. The agencies that regulate vaccines are continuously evaluating this balance. As new safety information emerges, it is included in the information in the leaflet that accompanies the vaccine. In the UK, there was no age restriction on the AstraZeneca COVID-19 vaccine initially. As reports of blood clots started to surface, the MHRA restricted the use of the vaccine to people aged thirty and over, as the risk from the disease below this age was slightly lower than the risk of a clot following the vaccine. This age cut-off was later raised to forty, again based on benefit versus risk. If the benefit risk equation changes significantly, the vaccine may be withdrawn altogether. This happened in 1992, when one of the MMR vaccines in use was shown to cause a mild form of meningitis, due to the strain of mumps that was in the vaccine. That mumps strain is no longer used.

There will always be concern about the safety of vaccines. At the moment, the pendulum has swung in their favour, as we are seeing the return of epidemics, and people realise that a few side effects is much better than the diseases. Despite the concerns that have been raised about the speed of development of COVID-19 vaccines, most people who are offered the vaccine are accepting it, as the risks of the disease are very real and present. In some countries, however, the tide is beginning to turn as the disease comes under control. Vaccination rates are flattening out and anti-vaccination protests are increasing. Myths are widespread: "it makes you infertile", "it alters your DNA"; both untrue.

As vaccine technology advances, we can look forward to vaccines with even fewer side effects. The introduction of new vaccines, especially if rolled out on mass scale, will, however, inevitably throw up more safety signals. In a utopian world all vaccines would have zero side effects, but this won't happen any time soon. We need to keep a perspective on the balance of benefit versus risk and not be lulled into a false sense of security when a vaccine gets a disease under control. Vaccines have become the victim of their own success, but when you balance the risk of vaccination versus the risk of not getting vaccinated, it's a no-brainer. Vaccines have side effects, but the alternative is much worse. I'm sure the vicar would agree.

10

Vaccines Don't Save Lives, Vaccination Does

According to the World Health Organization (WHO), vaccines prevent 2.5 million deaths a year, mostly in children. Another 1.5 million deaths could be prevented if all the vaccines available today were fully used. And that's not counting the impact of COVID-19 vaccines. The WHO also estimates that every year, 20 million children under the age of one still do not receive the most basic vaccines. Babies continue to die unnecessarily from whooping cough, measles, diphtheria and tetanus. Nearly all of these avoidable deaths are in the developing world. Stanley Plotkin, one of the world's leading vaccine experts, put this in context when he said that "only clean drinking water has had a greater impact on public health than vaccines". Today, 785 million people in the world still don't have clean drinking water, and there are over 1 million deaths a year due to contaminated water. Clean water and vaccination are the two most important public health interventions in the world.

The impact a vaccine has on death and disease depends on two things: the effectiveness of the vaccine and the number of people vaccinated. A vaccine with 100% efficacy has zero impact if no-one gets it. A vaccine with just 50% efficacy can have a big impact if 100% of people are vaccinated. A simple equation for this:

$$\text{Vaccine efficacy} \times \text{Vaccine coverage} = \text{Vaccine impact}$$

Eric Tayag, an epidemiologist who served as Health Secretary for the Philippines put it beautifully: "Vaccines don't save lives, vaccination does." Eric is an inspirational advocate for health promotion, who gets his messages across by dancing Gangnam-style (for the uniniti-ated, Gangnam is a high-energy Korean dance-pop tune that became a global craze in 2012); US President Barack Obama and British Prime Minster David Cameron were both afficionados.

Vaccines protect individuals, but also protect their contacts. Healthcare workers are prioritised to get vaccines for influenza and hepatitis B so they don't infect their patients. Boys are vaccinated against rubella (German measles) so that they don't pass the virus onto pregnant women. The impact of vaccines goes far beyond protecting individuals, as they can stop unvaccinated people catching the disease. This is due to herd immunity, which has become a bit of a hot topic since COVID-19 arrived. Let's look at this more closely. Imagine a town with a population of a 1,000. Nobody in the town is immune to disease X – they have never had the disease, and they have not been vaccinated against it. Someone with the disease comes into our imaginary town. Chances are the disease will spread like wildfire, and soon everyone will become infected. Now imagine the same town, but this time half of the people in the town are immune, either because they have had the disease or were vaccinated (or both). The disease will spread, but more slowly, as the person with the disease can only give it to the people who aren't immune. Now try it with ninety percent of the town being immune, from having caught the disease and/or getting vaccinated.

DOI: 10.1201/9781003303879-10

It is getting pretty difficult for the infectious person to find non-immune people. The person with the disease is only infectious for a short time, just a few days, so they might not bump into anyone who isn't immune in time to pass it on. The disease has nowhere to go and stops spreading. The ten percent of non-immune people have been spared by herd immunity. As long as they remain in their "herd" they are protected; however if they move to another town, where fewer people are immune, and the disease is still spreading, they can catch the disease.

Some infectious diseases are spread more easily than others. The more infectious a disease is, the higher the percentage of people that need to be immune, from the disease or vaccination, to reach herd immunity. The basic reproduction number (known as R_0 for short) is the term used to describe the infectiousness of a disease. Before the COVID-19 pandemic, the R number, as it has come to be known, was something that was only discussed in the obscure world inhabited by infectious disease epidemiologists and mathematical modellers. Now it is part of our daily vocabulary, so it's worth spending a bit of time understanding it properly. The R_0 is the number of people who will, on average, catch a disease from one infected person, in the situation where no-one is immune. Each infectious disease has a different R_0. Measles, with an R_0 of between twelve and eighteen, is top of the league. The original strain of COVID-19 had an R_0 of two to three, the Delta variant was between six and seven, and Omicron could be as high as ten. This is much higher than the flu (one to two). If the R_0 is less than one, the disease will no longer spread. Think back to our town of a 1,000 people in the scenario when no-one is immune. A disease with an R_0 of two will be able to spread quickly, as one case will give rise to two cases and each of those two cases will give rise to two more, and so on. But if you make it more difficult to spread, say by quarantining cases or wearing masks, then it becomes more difficult to spread. With strict enough measures you can bring the R_0 below one. If the R_0 now becomes say 0.9, ten people with the disease would only pass it on to nine people. Those nine would pass it on to eight (strictly speaking 8.1 but rounded down), and so on. The disease eventually dies out.

The R_0 is used by mathematical modellers to predict what will happen to a disease in different scenarios. Mathematical models are theoretical simulations of disease transmission. These models can be used to work out the impact of control measures such as reducing social contact, and also the percentage of people that need to be vaccinated to achieve herd immunity and stop the disease spreading. With increasing computer power, the number of scenarios that can be modelled is almost limitless. However, models are based on all kinds of assumptions; how many contacts each person has with other people and for how long, how long an infectious person stays infectious for, how long people live for, and so on. In reality, society is much more complicated. Teenagers mix more amongst themselves than older people do, Londoners behave differently to people from Scotland, Turkish people have different social habits to Chinese. Infectious diseases also behave differently over time; as COVID-19 has shown, viruses can mutate, causing variants which may be more (or less) infectious and dangerous. Someone with a weakened immune system may take longer to get rid of the virus than a healthy person. Getting the R_0 down through changing population behaviour has become the mantra for governments, but this calculation has many limitations, as society does not divide into neat predictable packages. Mathematical models are a useful tool, but are not the be all and end all. Knowing how much disease there is and where and how it is spreading is what counts.

When I was doing my public health training, I visited an institute that would turn my career on its head. The Northern Line in London rattles through Hampstead, Golders Green, past the Hendon Police College and the Royal Air Force Museum, and eventually reaches Colindale. I got off and turned right down Colindale Avenue, passing roads with names like Agar Grove and Pasteur Close. I was going to the Headquarters of the Public Health Laboratory Service, the PHLS. The PHLS was set up during World War II as a network of laboratories that could respond to a biological warfare attack. This was thought to be a very real threat; the government even conducted experiments with anthrax on the remote uninhabited Scottish island of Gruinard. In the summers of 1942 and 1943, sheep were placed in open pens then exposed to bombs dropped from a Vickers Wellington bomber plane, scattering anthrax spores across the island. The sheep started dying within days. The tests were abandoned as war drew to a close, but Gruinard was known for years as the Island of Death. It was only declared habitable in 1990 after 280 tons of formaldehyde, the same chemical used to make inactivated vaccines, were dumped on the island and the topsoil removed. The biological attack never happened, but when peace came the government decided to keep the PHLS, to monitor infectious diseases nationally. Every week, its laboratories, which were scattered across the country from Truro to Newcastle, would send their summary reports to HQ in Colindale for analysis and interpretation. The nerve centre of the PHLS was the CDSC – the Communicable Disease Surveillance Centre. The CDSC was a long single-story building with a red roof, known as the Pizza Hut. I stepped inside, and knew immediately this was where I wanted to work, where I *had* to work. Epidemiologists were poring over data coming from in the labs, but also from other sources – notifiable diseases from the National Statistics Office, GP reports and death certificates. As outbreaks were identified, a team would be sent to investigate, find the source and stop it. This was medical sleuthing and I loved it. But what really inspired me was the Director, Spence Galbraith. "The Boss" as he was affectionately known, was crippled by arthritis, with bushy eyebrows and a look that told you immediately that he couldn't be fooled by anyone or anything. He knew inside out the strengths and weaknesses of all the data that poured in. But above all, he was a great leader, who believed in his team and gave them extraordinary opportunities. Within a few weeks of joining the CDSC, he sent me to represent the UK at a WHO meeting on vaccination targets for Europe. It was held in Karlovy Vary, a spa town in what was at that time Czechoslovakia. On arrival, the meeting organiser, Sieghart Dittman, a tall, courteous East German from the WHO European office, asked me to be the meeting rapporteur (he presumably thought that being a native English speaker would compensate for my total lack of experience). Straight in at the deep end. It was my first taste of international public health, with epidemiologists from all over Europe debating what it would take to eliminate measles and congenital rubella (the catastrophic fetal damage caused by catching rubella, German measles, in pregnancy). There was simultaneous translation into French, Russian and Spanish (the WHO has six official languages – English, French, Spanish, Russian, Arabic and Chinese). It was also my first visit to an Eastern Bloc country. After the meeting, I spent a day in Prague walking around the city's spectacular architecture with deserted streets and empty shops. I felt like I was on a film set. This was several years before the collapse of the Berlin Wall, and the country was still firmly under the influence of the Soviet Union. In the evening, I had dinner with the other British delegate and two of the Russian translators. We dined in a spectacular restaurant, with vast ceilings, lavish murals and chandeliers. Apart from our table, the only other customers were two young Russian soldiers, Kalashnikovs slung casually over their chairs. Our highly Westernised Russian interpreters didn't take kindly to their presence. One of them, a charming but feisty woman, launched into a blistering attack on the continuing Russian occupation of the country. Her colleague provided simultaneous translation of her tirade at the soldiers. The restaurant staff were suddenly nowhere to be seen. I had visions of a promising career ending in a hail of gunfire. Fortunately, that didn't happen (the soldiers actually looked rather chaste at the dressing down) and I went back to Colindale realising how lucky I was to live in a free democracy. The report of that meeting got me my first publication in the *British Medical Journal*.

I spent fifteen years at the CDSC. It was an epidemiologist's dream. I investigated outbreaks of salmonella in baby milk, botulism in hazelnut yoghurt, Legionnaires' disease at the BBC and necrotising fasciitis, the flesh-eating bug. But what really grabbed my attention were the outbreaks that could be controlled by vaccination. Measles and whooping cough were still rife in the UK, and meningitis was on the increase. Not long after I arrived, Dr Galbraith decided I should spend some time at the US Centers for Disease Control and Prevention in Atlanta. I worked there for six months, in the immunisation division. The United States was on the brink of measles elimination, with vaccine coverage rates that put the UK to shame. I came back and set up a method to rapidly monitor vaccine coverage, with quarterly "name and shame" league tables, by district. I also did several more stints at the World Health Organization, which took me to their offices in Copenhagen and Geneva, and meetings in Warsaw, Budapest and Berlin. My most interesting WHO mission, however, was a major investigation into an outbreak of diphtheria in the ex-USSR. The public health services had collapsed following the breakup of the Soviet Union and vaccination rates were plummeting. Diphtheria, which had virtually been eliminated from the region, had returned with a vengeance. The epidemic exploded during the 1990s, causing over a 140,000 cases and 4,000 deaths. On my first visit to Moscow, the Russian Minister of Health invited me to vodka and caviar in his office (at nine am!); I declined politely. I visited laboratories, polyclinics and hospitals, where I saw first-hand the lack of modern laboratory equipment, shortages of vaccines and absence of basic training. I ended up writing a manual on diphtheria prevention and control, my first (and only) publication in Russian. The WHO subsequently invited a team of Russian microbiologists to the UK, to spend a fortnight at the PHLS diphtheria reference lab, learning the latest techniques. It was a great success. At the end of their visit, we went to dinner at a North London Greek restaurant. As we sat down, each of our Russian guests solemnly set a bottle of vodka and a bottle of brandy on the table to toast their hosts. This time I did not refuse.

Working at the CDSC, I came to understand exactly how infectious disease information is used to identify and control epidemics, and how to decide which vaccines are recommended. The first step is getting a really good handle on the impact of the disease. This sounds obvious, but isn't always straightforward. Each data source tells you something different. Laboratory reports tell you about people who get sick, go to the doctor and get a specimen taken. They are accurate, but only represent a very small tip of the iceberg. Many infectious diseases are notifiable, which means that a doctor who sees a case has to report it to the local public health department. The system of notifiable diseases started in the UK in 1889, and continues today. There are currently thirty-three diseases on the list, including COVID-19. However, notifications don't usually need laboratory confirmation, so they may not be accurate. It can be difficult to tell a case of measles from a case of rubella without taking a sample to verify the diagnosis. Information on deaths tells you how severe a disease is, but represents an even smaller tip of the iceberg. There are different ways to decide whether a death was actually the cause of an infectious disease. This has been a big bone of contention in the COVID-19 pandemic; some countries count all deaths within a specified period of having a positive test, others only include deaths where COVID-19 is considered to be the direct cause of death. At the other end of the spectrum, mild cases, or cases without symptoms are at the bottom of the iceberg and are not usually picked up by any routine surveillance system.

I worked a lot on meningitis at the CDSC. It seems that it would be obvious to figure out the disease burden for such a well-known and serious illness. It's not that simple. Meningitis – inflammation of the lining of the brain – is a broad term that covers a whole range of illnesses from mild cases or even cases without symptoms, through to the most dramatic, fatal cases. It is caused by all kinds of viruses, for example mumps, as well as bacteria and sometimes fungi. There are several types of bacterial meningitis, many of which can only be distinguished from each other by a lab test. Doctors often give antibiotics when they suspect a case, which makes lab diagnosis very difficult, as the antibiotic kills the bacteria, so they cannot be grown in culture. Sometimes the meningitis bacteria don't cause meningitis at all, but instead they cause septicae-mia (blood poisoning), arthritis or even conjunctivitis. COVID-19 has exposed the minefield of interpreting infectious disease data. Sadly, the CDSC no longer exists (it was disbanded dur-ing a reorganisation of public health services). It was a unique hothouse of highly trained public health doctors, epidemiologists and statisticians. I sometimes wonder if the UK would have reacted sooner to the pandemic if Dr Galbraith's team of medical sleuths were still around.

While working at the CDSC, I became involved in figuring out how to plan a vaccination programme. Some diseases are easier to control than others. Before planning a vaccination programme, you need to think about what is realistically achievable. Do you simply want to reduce the number of cases to a manageable level, or eliminate the disease completely? Or even go one step further – eradication, meaning the organism doesn't exist anymore? Keeping a dis-ease under control is much easier than eliminating or eradicating it. This is where you need to know your enemy. Some diseases are quite simply too cunning to be mastered by vaccination. Others are rather more obliging. I have a check list of the ideal disease, which makes it amenable to be controlled by vaccination. I'm will look at these characteristics in detail.

Firstly, the disease needs to be difficult to transmit, with a low R_0. Vaccinating a community has the effect of reducing the R_0, and once you get the R_0 below one, the disease stops circulating. The closer the pre-vaccination R_0 is to one, the quicker you will get there with vaccination. Measles, with an R_0 of twelve to eighteen, is the most difficult to control. You need to vaccinate at least 95% of children in any given country to keep it in check. This is why there are measles outbreaks even when vaccine coverage is high. Polio has a rather lower R_0, five to seven, making it a more suitable candidate for eradication.

A second useful attribute for a disease is being confined to humans. Vaccinating against a disease that oscillates between animals and humans is like pushing water uphill. Flu is the classic example; every year, new strains emerge in animals, often birds, then spill over into humans. The ability of flu viruses to continually change, either incrementally (antigenic drift) or in big steps (antigenic shift) make them even less vaccine friendly. COVID-19 has the same ability to mutate, though rather more slowly than flu.

A less obvious disease characteristic is that it is easy to diagnose, and better still, easy to know who is immune. This is one of the reasons that made smallpox eradication feasible. The small-pox rash was be recognised immediately, and cases quarantined while their contacts were vac-cinated. Smallpox vaccination leaves an obvious scar, so village health workers could check people's immune status in seconds.

Finally, immunity to both the disease and the vaccine should be lifelong, so you don't have to keep revaccinating.

Going through my checklist, COVID-19 is far from the ideal disease, particularly as the newer variants have a higher R_0. I suspect that keeping the disease under control will be the objective for the foreseeable future.

As well as the ideal disease, you obviously need the ideal vaccine. An ideal vaccine would have 100% efficacy after one dose, no side effects, resistance to heat and freezing, protection against transmission as well as disease, provide lifelong immunity for everyone, and be admin-istrable by mouth or nasal spray. The ideal vaccine doesn't exist; polio is probably the closest thing.

To decide who should get vaccinated, you need to know who is most at risk. If everyone, or everyone in one age group is at risk, then it has to be a universal vaccination recommendation. The infectious diseases of children like measles and whooping cough are all indiscriminate, so vaccine recommendations apply to all children (unless they have a condition which means they can't be given the vaccine). Other diseases are more selective and infect only people who are at risk because of their job. For example, anthrax is a disease that affects people who are in close contact with untreated animal hides, like abattoir workers. Other vaccines like typhoid and hepatitis A are only given to people when they travel to countries where the diseases are common. Influenza affects everyone but is more serious in people with underlying health conditions, so flu vaccine policy is a mixture of universal recommendations for children and older people and selective recommendations for high-risk groups like people with chronic bronchitis, and pregnant women. Selective vaccination policies can be attractive to governments because they are less expensive, but they have drawbacks. When the UK first introduced rubella (German measles) vaccine, the government decided it should just be given to people at risk, namely, women of child-bearing age. Rubella is a relatively mild disease except in pregnancy, when it causes catastrophic effects on the developing fetus. Babies with congenital rubella syndrome are born deaf, with cataracts, heart defects and other irreversible complications. At the time, focusing on vaccinating women of child-bearing age seemed like a sensible approach; however, it became clear over time that it was going to be impossible to eliminate congenital rubella syndrome. The disease continued to circulate among boys and younger girls; inevitably some women didn't get vaccinated and would catch it while they were pregnant. In 1988, the UK policy changed to mass vaccination of all young children. The year before the policy switch there were 160 cases of congenital rubella syndrome; in 2003, there was just one. A similar debate is now happening with human papillomavirus (HPV), the cause of cervical cancer. Some countries vaccinate boys and girls; others just offer the vaccine to teenage girls. More and more countries are switching to vaccination of boys and girls. In the long run, universal vaccination is often the simpler and more effective option.

Health economics is also important. No country has a limitless health budget, so when a new vaccine comes along, the government must decide whether or not to prioritise it. This is a poisoned chalice. It's easy enough to work out the cost of a vaccination programme, but what price do you put on someone who dies, or has a lifelong disability because they didn't get vaccinated? Health economists try to take this into account by measuring quality of life, the duration of illness and disability, health service utilisation and so on, but inevitably there is an element of subjectivity. If you just take the healthcare costs into account, the return on investment doesn't look nearly as good as if you include the wider costs. For example, when a child gets chickenpox, they will be off school for a week or two, so one of the parents has to stay at home, which impacts their economic productivity. The child will then give it to their siblings, so the cycle is repeated. Most of the economic benefit of chickenpox vaccination is preventing these indirect costs. Luckily, most vaccines are relatively inexpensive, so health economic analyses are usually positive. Wealthier countries will usually adopt a new vaccine sooner or later, but it can take many years for some vaccines to get into the national vaccination calendar. In the UK, the only vaccine that has not yet been recommended for all children is chickenpox. On the other hand, the UK was the first country in the world to recommend meningitis vaccine for all babies; this is because the UK had one of the highest rates of disease in the developed world.

Vaccination also has economic benefits beyond the impact on individuals. David Bloom, an American economist, makes the point that a society that controls infectious diseases by vaccination is more productive and economically more successful. Women have fewer babies, as they can be confident that their children will survive, so find it easier to go to work. There are fewer handicapped children that require state support. Children that don't get infectious diseases because they are vaccinated do better at school, and become more economically productive.

There is inevitably a political element in vaccine policy. Some diseases attract more attention than others. Meningitis is relatively uncommon but very scary and headline worthy. Vaccination has an immediate impact on meningitis, and is likely to be more attractive from a government's point of view than a chronic disease, like hepatitis B, where the long-term effects of the disease are only seen after many years. It takes twenty years to see the full impact of a hepatitis B vaccination programme; well beyond the lifespan of most governments. Health economists actually take this into account using something called discounting, where disease impact that occurs in the future has a lower monetary value than something that happens immediately. With the COVID-19 pandemic, health economics has taken a bit of a back seat. Governments have poured money into COVID-19 vaccines at an unprecedented rate. As the disease comes under control, health economics is starting to play a role in the deciding the frequency of boosters and whether to extend the vaccine to younger children.

Once a government has decided to introduce a new vaccine, they need to work out an implementation plan. Most health services are working at full stretch, so adding a new activity, especially if it applies to everyone, puts yet more strain on the system. Most vaccines are given by general practitioners, nurses, paediatricians and sometimes in pharmacies; however, it may sometimes be logistically easier to give them in schools, colleges or the workplace. The COVID-19 roll out has created all kinds of innovative vaccination centres. My brother-in-law was very chuffed to get his vaccine at Lord's Cricket Ground. Some countries have employed vets to give vaccines.

Various tactics have been developed to get people vaccinated, including incentives for doctors to give vaccines, and sanctions for people who don't get vaccinated. Many countries, like the United States, have laws requiring children to be vaccinated before they go to school or go to college. These are effective, but people can be exempt from the law if they object on religious or philosophical grounds. Some US states have closed this loophole which was being increasingly used by people opposed to vaccination. Vaccine laws are controversial and set up a debate about individual liberty versus collective responsibility. Should vaccination be compulsory to protect vulnerable people who cannot be vaccinated? The debate has become much more edgy with COVID-19, with countries adopting various stick-and-carrot techniques to boost vaccination rates.

During a WHO meeting on polio, somebody asked the question: "What is the biggest obstacle to polio eradication?" Rafe Henderson, the head of the WHO Immunisation Programme grabbed the mic and replied "bad leadership". Laws and incentives are good tools to boost vaccination rates, but the most important factor is strong leadership of the programme. Look at South America. Some of the poorest people in the world live there. Imagine the logistics of getting vaccines to remote tribes in the Amazon. There is guerrilla warfare, dictatorship and stagnating economies. Yet this was the first region in the world to eradicate polio. The first region to eliminate measles. The swing factor was one person. Ciro de Quadros, a diminutive Brazilian with a neat grey beard and a permanent grin, worked at the Pan American Health Organization (PAHO). PAHO is the branch of the World Health Organization for North and South America. I met him a few times. He exuded passion and optimism, which was highly infectious. He persuaded governments of the importance of vaccination, visited remote Amazonian tribes, negotiated truces with terrorist organisations so campaigns could be carried out safely, raised money and inspired everyone that had anything to do with vaccines. The earlier eradication of smallpox was also due to a great leader. Donald Ainslie Henderson – "DA" – led the WHO effort to eradicate the disease for ten years. He was a truly charismatic figure who created a vision for what needed to be done, and followed it to the end.

No matter how robust a vaccine programme is, it can be unravelled overnight with misinformation. Type "vaccination" into Google, and you will be directed to a galaxy of websites; good, bad and seriously ugly. There is no shortage of misinformation about COVID-19 vaccines, ranging from vaguely plausible but misguided theories (e.g., herd immunity from the disease is better than vaccination) to the downright silly (Bill Gates is going to control the world by inserting traceable microchips into the vaccine). A swathe of anti-vaccination books is starting to appear.

After a vaccine programme has been implemented, it is vital to track its progress. A vaccine that has performed beautifully in clinical trials may not look quite so good in the real world of delayed or missed appointments, temperature deviations and incorrectly administered vaccines. The immunity might wane over time, or be better than expected. The disease can change as transmission patterns are interrupted. As these real-world data emerge, tweaks are sometimes needed. The schedule for the meningitis C vaccines in the UK has changed several times over the last twenty years, with progressively fewer doses, and the vaccine being given later in childhood. No-one knows how COVID-19 will pan out; most countries have given a third dose and many are now recommending a fourth dose as the virus continues to mutate and immunity wanes.

Monitoring vaccine coverage in real time is equally important. Rates can plummet overnight in response to a scare, and campaigns need to be mounted to avert the return of epidemics.

Most decision-making for vaccines happens at the national level. There is typically an independent expert committee which advises the government who then decides. The committee usually includes specialists in infectious diseases, immunologists, paediatricians, general practitioners, and sometimes, laypeople. The UK committee is called the Joint Committee on Vaccination and Immunization (JCVI); the US equivalent is the Advisory Committee on Immunisation Practices (ACIP). In some countries, decisions are made at the subnational level, for example in Spain which has seventeen autonomous regions, each deciding its own policy. This sounds chaotic, but in practice, the recommendations are very similar everywhere. As well as deciding policy, governments often also buy vaccines directly from manufacturers and distribute them to vaccination centres, keeping the cost down as they purchase in bulk. This strategy has been widely adopted for COVID-19 vaccines.

There are a few multinational players worth mentioning. The World Health Organization is a branch of the United Nations, with its HQ based in Geneva. My father, also a public health doctor (and also called Norman!) worked there (he was the head for Europe), so I suppose I have inherited some of his genes. The WHO's strength lies in its collective membership of 194 member states. A WHO recommendation is a global mandate for action and has been particularly successful for vaccines. Smallpox would not have been eradicated without the WHO. Polio eradication is close. The WHO cannot force countries to act, but its recommendations are hard to ignore.

The United Nations Children's Fund, better known as UNICEF, is another agency of the United Nations that has a vital role in vaccination. Based in New York, its mission is to provide humanitarian aid to children worldwide. UNICEF works in the field, getting vaccines to children in the poorest countries of the world. UNICEF receives money from governments but raises a lot of its money from charitable donations and the fundraising efforts of an army of volunteers. When you buy one of their Christmas cards you are helping vaccinate children in Africa. I helped organise a rock concert for UNICEF when I worked for GlaxoSmithKline in Belgium, featuring the company's musical talent.

It would be impossible to talk about vaccines without mentioning Bill Gates. Over the last twenty years, the founder of Microsoft has donated several billion dollars to vaccine research and development through his charity, the Bill and Melinda Gates Foundation. His main priority is diseases of the developing world; he financed much of the development of the world's first malaria vaccine which is now being rolled out in Africa. I met him when he came to visit GlaxoSmithKline's vaccine HQ in Belgium. He looks for all the world like a geeky schoolboy, and boy does he know his stuff. It was clear from his answers to our questions that he has an encyclopaedic knowledge of vaccines. He was also the driving force between setting up a coalition called GAVI, the Global Alliance for Vaccines and Immunisation (now simply called the Vaccine Alliance), between the WHO, UNICEF and the World Bank. GAVI helps the poorest countries of the world implement vaccination programmes. It's not a free lunch; to be eligible for GAVI support, a country has to be able to show they are capable of running a sustainable programme, they pay for some of the cost, and are expected to take over the full cost in the long term. GAVI has massive purchasing power, which keeps the cost down. Half of the world's children are vaccinated with GAVI support. The COVID-19 pandemic has created more multinational vaccination efforts, such as COVAX, the WHO-led initiative to ensure less well-off countries get access to vaccines. CEPI, the Coalition for Epidemic Preparedness Innovations is another multinational organisation that has played a role in coordinating the global response to the pandemic

I'd like to talk a bit about the vaccine industry. In Chapter 8, I discussed how the complexity of manufacture means that there are relatively few companies that are able to manufacture vaccines on a global scale. The reality is that there is not enough capacity to manufacture all the recommended vaccines for everyone in the world, let alone COVID-19. More and more vaccines are being developed, the world's population is growing and ageing, and new diseases are emerging. For now, demand outstrips supply. This places a huge responsibility on the companies that have the wherewithal to meet this demand. The behaviour of the pharmaceutical industry has often been criticised for unfair pricing, unsubstantiated claims and unethical research. There is no doubt that some of this is justified, however, the world of vaccines is a bit different. Most vaccines are sold to governments and supranational organisations, often with very low profit. Oral polio vaccine is currently sold to UNICEF at ¢12–19 (US) per dose. The most expensive childhood vaccine, which protects against thirteen strains of pneumococcal disease, goes to UNICEF for $2.90 a dose. The US government pays $150 a dose for the same vaccine. Companies that make vaccines often have a tiered pricing system, where the price is linked to a country's ability to pay. Much of the profit that comes from the higher price countries like the US goes back into developing new vaccines. In some countries the company will partner with a local manufacturer, either as a joint venture, or by progressively transferring the technology so that they can become fully independent to make vaccines themselves. A good example is the partnership between GlaxoSmithKline and the Oswaldo Cruz Foundation (Fiocruz) in Brazil. Fiocruz has existed as a national public health institute in Brazil since the nineteenth century. Technology transfers agreements between GlaxoSmithKline and Fiocruz have enabled Brazil to become self-sufficient in MMR, rotavirus, *Haemophilus influenzae* type b (Hib) and pneumococcal vaccines. In 2020, GlaxoSmithKline teamed up with Sanofi Pasteur, a major competitor, to develop a vaccine for COVID-19. The Serum Institute of India is making the Oxford/AstraZeneca vaccine for the Indian population. AstraZeneca provides the know-how; the Serum Institute has the manufacturing capacity (measured by volume, they are the biggest manufacturer of vaccines in the world).

The vaccine industry is not perfect, but my experience of working there was very positive. From the top down, there was a genuine drive to do good for public health. Many of the people there, especially in research, have a background in public health and have worked in developing countries. Diseases of the developing world are a high priority – vaccines for malaria, dengue fever and tuberculosis have all come from the multinational vaccine companies in the last few years.

Although most vaccines have been developed by the big multinationals, there are exceptions. For more than a century, epidemics of meningitis have swept across sub-Saharan Africa. The epidemics start in January, as hot dry winds blow sand southwards from the Sahara Desert, and stop abruptly when the rains arrive, usually in June. The so-called meningitis belt has the highest incidence of the disease in the world by far. Nearly all of the cases are caused by one strain of the meningitis bacterium, group A. The Meningitis Vaccine Project was established in 2001 with funding from Bill Gates, to develop a vaccine specifically for the meningitis belt. This is a partnership between WHO and PATH (Programme for Appropriate Technology in Health). The vaccine, which is manufactured by the Serum Institute of India, reduced the rate of disease by ninety-four percent, and in countries that have conducted mass vaccination campaigns, the disease has all but disappeared. The meningitis belt vaccine – MenAfrivac – sells for under ¢50 a dose.

The COVID-19 pandemic has provided a massive boost to vaccine development. Companies like Sinopharm and Sinovac in China and Bharat Biotech in India, which until now focused on their own domestic markets, are licensing their vaccines in Europe, the Middle East and South America. Moderna and Novavax had never taken a vaccine all the way to licensure before the pandemic. Their success with COVID-19 will be a huge boost to the other vaccines in their pipelines. One of the few positive legacies of the pandemic will be a revitalised vaccine industry with new players and new technologies. More of this in Chapter 11.

Over the last decade a new phrase has entered the language of vaccines. Vaccine hesitancy describes why people choose not to be vaccinated or to have their children vaccinated. Vaccine hesitancy covers a spectrum, from people who are slightly unsure to those who downright and publicly oppose all vaccines. The phrase might be new but opposition to vaccination is not. When smallpox vaccination became compulsory in nineteenth century England, protests erupted, often violently. Copies of laws were burned in public, and an effigy of Edward Jenner was lynched. Nowhere was the anti-vaccination movement more strident than in Leicester, where the authorities were particularly tough on people who refused to be vaccinated. In 1884, 3,000 people were prosecuted and fined ten shillings or sent to jail for seven days. Police collecting a fine from one Arthur Ward threatened his pregnant wife with prison. The argument sent her into premature labour and the child was stillborn. The following year, there was a mass protest in the city. Although largely peaceful, the scale of the demonstration sent shock waves through the establishment. In 1889, a law was passed allowing conscientious objection to vaccination, and eventually the legislation was repealed altogether.

There are many reasons why people are hesitant about vaccines. Worries about side effects, overloading the immune system, ingredients in the vaccine, and religious beliefs provide ample reasons to delay or avoid vaccination. The world's leading expert on vaccine hesitancy is Heidi Larson, an American anthropologist, based at the London School of Hygiene and Tropical Medicine. She runs the Vaccine Confidence Project, which tracks why people hesitate to vaccinate, all over the world. It turns out that confidence in vaccines is lowest in Europe, with France at the bottom of the league table (although when push comes to shove, most French people have accepted the COVID-19 vaccine). In a brilliant TED Talk, she explains why vaccination is singled out for such a crisis in confidence. (A TED Talk is a fifteen-minute inspirational talk, which can be on any subject, with the slogan "ideas worth spreading".) Most vaccination programmes are driven by governments and most vaccines are produced by multinational pharmaceutical companies. Both feature a long way down the list of whom people trust. The benefits of vaccination are usually championed by experts – paediatricians, infectious disease epidemiologists, mathematical modellers, who are remote, unrelatable figures. Bad science underpins the anti-vaccination movement, and social media provides a limitless platform for misinformation, which is exploited much more effectively by the antivaccine lobby than by the pro-vaccinators. And perhaps most importantly, vaccination is for everyone. A perfect scapegoat.

Professor Larson argues, and I agree with her, that the basic problem is not one of lack of information but of lack of trust. She advocates changing the paradigm, to de-medicalise how we communicate information about vaccines. For example, invite parents who have gone through the experience of vaccinating their children, to provide online chat support to parents with concerns. We should also listen to people who oppose vaccines, not demonise them. I have a friend who chose to not get her children vaccinated with MMR (although, haphazardly, they have had some vaccines). She is a highly intelligent maths teacher, who loves and deeply cares about her children. She did what she thought was best for them. I may not agree, but telling her she's stupid or irresponsible is neither respectful nor helpful.

Getting vaccines to all who need them is still a massive challenge. The WHO has an ambitious goal to ensure that everyone, at every age, gets the full possible benefit from vaccines by 2030. Rapid manufacturing, digital technology, and innovative delivery systems can make this happen. There is political will for the necessary investment, at least for now. Vaccination will save millions more lives.

11

Rocket Science

On March 16, 2020, Jennifer Haller, a fifty-three-year-old operations manager at a Seattle tech company, became the first person in the world to be injected with an experimental COVID-19 vaccine. This happened just sixty-five days after Professor Zhang Yongzhen from the Shanghai Public Health Clinical Centre published the genetic sequence of the virus. He had worked forty hours, round the clock, to map its full genome. A mere 269 days after the start of the trial, Margaret Keenan, an Irish grandmother from Coventry, was the first person to receive an approved COVID-19 vaccine. "It was my best early birthday present" (she turned ninety-one a few days later). Even a decade ago, this timetable would have been unthinkable; it typically takes up to ten years to develop a new vaccine. At the time of writing, there are 196 COVID-19 vaccines in development, and thirty-eight have been approved. Some of these are traditional vaccines but the majority are using technology that has been developed in the twenty-first century.

The ability to develop and manufacture new vaccines is advancing at a breath-taking speed. Viruses can be manipulated at ease; bacterial proteins can be manufactured to order; genetic sequences are published online. The science is evolving daily.

The modern era of vaccines began in 1986, when scientists at the Universities of California and Washington, and the Chiron Corporation, developed the first genetically engineered vaccine, hepatitis B. A few years later, the same technology would be used to produce a vaccine for human papillomavirus, the cause of cancer of the cervix. It was however the emergence of new epidemics – Ebola, SARS, MERS – that created the impetus for gene-based vaccines to realise their potential. When the COVID-19 pandemic hit, research into these vaccines was already well advanced. One gene-based pandemic vaccine – for Ebola – had already been used in 2015 to successfully quell an epidemic in Guinea, West Africa. Unravelling the genome – all the genetic information about an organism – has been a game-changer for vaccine science.

The success of gene-based COVID-19 vaccines is nothing short of spectacular. In the early days of the pandemic, a group of scientists analysed the rate of success of vaccines for new and emerging diseases during the previous fifteen years, success being defined as getting from a Phase 2 clinical trial through to being approved for use. The success rate was ten percent. Based on this, not even the most optimistic person would have predicted that so many COVID-19 vaccines would reach the approval milestone, within one year, with such high protection rates. The first four vaccines to be approved in the United States and Europe – Pfizer, Moderna, Oxford/AstraZeneca, Johnson & Johnson – all use gene-based technology; the Russian Sputnik V vaccine is also gene-based. Not all gene-based COVID-19 vaccines have succeeded (Merck and the Pasteur Institute both abandoned their programmes); however, genetic vaccines are now firmly established in the premier division. What these modern vaccines have shown is that when a new disease appears, a vaccine can be constructed within days. This will transform the way the world responds to epidemics. As humans encroach further and further into the natural world, we will need more vaccines for diseases we haven't yet encountered and those we don't even yet know about. Bill Gates gave a stark warning about future pandemics in a 2015 TED Talk. He said "we are not ready for the next pandemic." Seventy years earlier, Albert Camus, the French-Algerian

DOI: 10.1201/9781003303879-11

philosopher and author wrote a book about the plague in which he said, "there have been as many plagues as wars in history, yet always plagues and wars take people equally by surprise."

Over the last few years, gene-based science has created platforms that enable new vaccines to be made to order. The success of gene-based COVID-19 vaccines has paved the way for vaccines not just for pandemics, but for other diseases that have hitherto eluded conventional approaches, such as HIV. Gene-based vaccines are in development for Lassa fever (a viral disease that causes internal bleeding, like Ebola, which has caused outbreaks in West Africa since the 1950s) and for Zika virus, the mosquito-borne disease which has recently spread from Africa to many regions, especially South America. Zika virus causes devastating damage to the unborn baby if caught in pregnancy; the baby is born with a small head (microcephaly) and severe mental retardation. Gene-based vaccines are being pursued for respiratory syncytial virus (RSV), which causes a serious respiratory illness in young children and the elderly, and for cytomegalovirus (CMV), anther illness which causes damage to the developing fetus in pregnant women; one in 200 pregnancies are affected by CMV. A trial of an RNA vaccine against Epstein-Barr virus (EBV) has started. EBV is the cause of infectious mononucleosis (better known as glandular fever) but has also been linked to multiple sclerosis. Influenza vaccines will likely be improved by using gene-based technology. The world of viral vaccines is being revolutionised as the genomes of these tiny organisms are laid bare.

While vaccines continue to conquer infectious diseases, a whole new category of vaccines is in its infancy; therapeutic vaccines. Traditional vaccines work by preventing infectious diseases, whereas therapeutic vaccines are given to treat people who already have the disease. They work by stimulating your immune system to help you fight the disease. There are now a whole host of therapeutic vaccines at different stages of development. These vaccines don't just target infectious diseases, they also have the potential to be used for a whole range of cancers. Therapeutic cancer vaccines contain cancer cells or cells from the immune system, which have either been taken from the person with the disease, or grown in a lab. To date there are only two approved cancer vaccines: one for prostate cancer, and one for bladder cancer (which actually uses the same components as BCG, the vaccine for tuberculosis). There are therapeutic vaccines now being developed for cancer of the cervix, breast, lung, pancreas and others. These custom-made, personalised vaccines will shape the future of cancer treatment, and have given medicine a new word: immunotherapy (also called immuno-oncology). Therapeutic vaccines for infectious diseases are being developed for those that become chronic, such as hepatitis B and HIV. Many of the therapeutic vaccines in development also rely on gene-based technology.

Despite the advantages of gene-based vaccines, the ability to manufacture at scale is still a rate-limiting step. There are some novel approaches being used to tackle this. A Canadian biotech company, Medicago, is using plants as the vehicle for production of its COVID-19 vaccine. The genetic material of the virus is inserted into a bacterium, which is then used to infect *Nicotiana benthamiana*, a close relative of the tobacco plant. The plant acts as a natural bioreactor, churning out the spike protein component of COVID-19 in vast quantities. It takes about a week. The company hopes to be able to make up to a billion doses a year once the technology is fully up and running. Another company that I am now working with, SpyBiotech, based in Oxford, has developed a type of bacterial superglue, which can be used to bind together components of vaccines in a much more effective way, enabling new vaccines to be developed more rapidly. These new technologies are highly adaptable and can be rapidly applied to new diseases, or disease variants.

While lab scientists are getting smarter at manipulating genetic material and proteins, computers are starting to play a significant role in vaccine development. During the 1990s, scientists began to sequence the entire genome of microorganisms. Rino Rappuoli, an Italian researcher from Siena, saw the potential for vaccines. A quiet unassuming man, Rino is a giant in the field of vaccine discovery. He invented reverse vaccinology, which uses bioinformatics (the methods and software needed to understand biological data) to design new vaccines. With the entire sequence of a microorganism sitting on a computer, it can be scanned to look for potential components that could go into a vaccine. This is much quicker than the traditional hit or miss approach, where multiple different candidates are produced, in the hope that one succeeds. Rino used this to develop the first successful vaccine against meningococcal group B vaccine. He found over 600 possible component antigens, eventually incorporating the four most common ones into the vaccine. The age of computer-designed vaccines had arrived.

As well as speeding up basic research, information technology will transform the way clinical trials are run and vaccines are monitored once they are approved. Information about volunteers in a vaccine trial will be linked to their personal health data, which can be used to track the effect of the vaccine in a much more detailed and sophisticated way than at present. It will be easier to identify, and contact people who would be suitable volunteers to participate in clinical trials. This might sound rather like big brother watching you, but we already live in a world where your shopping, reading and viewing preferences are known and used to target people with personalised messages. There could be substantial benefits from using IT to streamline research. As information from the trial will accumulate more rapidly, side effects could be detected sooner, and conclusions about the vaccine's effect will be known earlier. When trials are over and the vaccine is approved and rolled out, information on people who received the vaccine can be used to check its real-world effectiveness and safety. If there is an issue with a particular vaccine batch, this could be spotted more quickly.

One of the biggest nuts to crack is the ability of vaccines to withstand temperature changes. If vaccines could be shipped around the world without having to be kept within a narrow temperature range, it would transform the supply chain. In 2018, the WHO approved a thermostable vaccine for rotavirus, the major cause of childhood diarrhoea, developed by the Serum Institute of India. Some of the COVID-19 vaccines being developed are heat stable, and will not need to be stored in a fridge. There will be more heat stable vaccines in the future. Even if these vaccines are more expensive, the savings from the supply chain logistics would be worth it. Vaccines could be transported around the world and stored without cold boxes or fridges. Fewer vaccine doses would be wasted, as there would no temperature deviations. It would be much easier to set up mass vaccination clinics without having to think about cold storage. This would have a huge impact in developing countries, particularly in remote areas.

Another big area of research is needle-free vaccination. Decades of work are at last starting to bear fruit. There is already one flu vaccine which is injected by a high-pressure jet of liquid. It takes a tenth of a second and is painless. There are several trials ongoing of skin patches, which deliver the vaccine through hundreds of tiny microneedles, each one no thicker than a human hair. The patches are like an Elastoplast, which is applied to the skin, then peeled off after the vaccine has penetrated the skin, rather like a nicotine patch. In November 2020, a group of researchers from Connecticut published the results of a study in rats in which they applied a skin patch loaded with microneedles containing an approved human pneumococcal vaccine. The rats had no side effects from the patch, and the immune responses were high – equivalent to giving multiple doses of the vaccine by injection. These findings have to be confirmed in human studies, but it is likely that needle-free vaccines will be here in a few years.

Another needle-free route is vaccines which are given by nasal spray. The lining of your nose is rich with immune cells, so when you squirt a vaccine up the nose, the immune response kicks into action immediately. Nasal spray vaccines have an important advantage for diseases that are spread by the respiratory route. A vaccine that is injected into a muscle provides a good immune response in the blood stream, but the immune response on the lining of your nose and throat is often weaker. When you catch a respiratory virus, it first grows on these upper airways, so a nasally administered vaccine that has a strong first line of defence can stop this happening before it goes any further. There is currently only one approved nasal vaccine, for influenza, but others are in development (one of the new COVID-19 vaccines being developed is a nasal vaccine).

Notwithstanding these promising advances, it will be many years before needles can be replaced by patches and sprays, and most vaccines are likely to be injected for the foreseeable future.

The development of COVID-19 vaccines represents a scientific effort that is unparalleled in human history. Thousands of scientists around the world have focused on one virus. Armies of virologists are sequencing the virus on a daily basis, discovering new variants and building up a huge database which will allow the vaccine to be adapted and improved. Laboratories have sprung up all over the world, discovering new techniques to test for the virus and for immunity. Infectious disease epidemiologists, mathematical modellers, and behavioural scientists have refined how we track and predict the course of the epidemic. The network of clinical trial centres has mushroomed, expanding the global capacity to conduct trials. Advances in manufacturing techniques have enabled RNA and DNA vaccines to be produced at massive scale, for the first time. Biotech companies are investing massively in new platforms, and investors have discovered that vaccines are a good bet. A whole new generation of scientists are hungry to work on vaccines. This will have a lasting impact that will go far beyond COVID-19. Now that's rocket science.

A-to-Z of Vaccines

There are thousands of bacteria and viruses that can inhabit us humans. Most are harmless; some are even helpful, like the ones that help digest your food. It's a relatively elite band that make us ill enough to merit the slog of developing and making a vaccine. I'm going to introduce you to these villains and the vaccines against them. You will have had many of them at some time in your life. Some are rather exotic, and you will probably never need the vaccine. For the bacterial infections, I've thrown in their Latin names (in italics according to scientific convention), I think they sound so much better than in English. Sadly, the Latin names for viruses sound less grand (the spoilsports who run the classification system for viruses have decreed the names should be as short as possible). Vaccine recommendations change regularly, so you should always check with your health provider.

Anthrax

Definitely in the exotic category, this is a bacterial infection caused by a hardy creature called *Bacillus anthracis*. It has the rather annoying ability of being able to form spores – a tough version of itself that can lie dormant, sometimes for years, only to wake up and wreak havoc when it gets into a human. Anthrax is common in vegetarian animals like cows and sheep, and the spores survive in their by-products like skin, hides, wool and bone meal. The spores also hibernate happily in soil. Humans usually catch the disease by skin contact, but sometimes by inhaling or swallowing the spores. Anthrax is very, very rare, and only affects people who have regular close contact with animal products, like slaughtermen, butchers or people who work with leather. There have been a few cases in injecting drug users, from heroin that was contaminated with spores. Because of its dormant state, anthrax has been used as a biological weapon. In September 2001, just after 9/11, several letters containing anthrax spores were sent to US news media offices and two senators, causing five deaths and another seventeen infections.

The vaccine is inactivated. You need four injections to be protected, and if you are at long-term risk of exposure you may need a booster every ten years. The vaccine often causes a local reaction, and sometimes fever. You only really need to be vaccinated if you are likely to have direct contact with the spores, for example in a laboratory working on the bacterium.

Cholera

Nowadays, you probably only hear about cholera when an outbreak is reported in a refugee camp somewhere in Africa. In fact, it is quite common throughout Asia and Africa, thriving in conditions of poor sanitation. It also has the dubious honour of belonging to the elite group of infectious diseases that cause pandemics (global epidemics). The other members of the pandemic club are influenza, plague, HIV and COVID-19. Over the last two centuries, there have been seven cholera pandemics; the seventh pandemic lasted from 1961 to 1975, affecting countries in Asia, South America, the Middle East and parts of Europe. The agent responsible is *Vibrio cholerae*, a bacterium that looks like a comma under the microscope, and is spread by contaminated water. If you want to discover more about cholera, I can highly recommend a visit to the John Snow pub, in London. John Snow was a doctor who specialised in anaesthetics, but was also interested in cholera. He worked out that it was a waterborne disease, scotching the widely held "miasma" theory that diseases like plague and cholera were spread by noxious air emanating from rotting organic matter. In the summer of 1854, an outbreak of cholera in the centre of London gave him the opportunity to prove his theory. He plotted all the cases on a map. They were clustered around Broad Street in Soho, which was the site of a public water pump. Snow persuaded the sceptical council to remove the handle of the pump, bringing the outbreak to an end. During his meticulous investigation, he identified a case in a widow who lived in what is now West Hampstead, several miles from Broad Street. She had her water delivered from the Broad Street pump because she preferred the taste. Her last delivery was on August 31; she died two days later from cholera. The John Snow pub stands on the site of the pump (it's now called Broadwick Street). You can enjoy a pint and read about one of the most famous outbreak investigations in history. If this whets your appetite for more, £15 will buy a life membership of the John Snow Society, with an invitation to the annual pump handle lecture held at the nearby London School of Tropical Medicine and Hygiene. Dr Anthony Fauci delivered the 2021 pump handle lecture, eighty years old and sharp as a tack.

Cholera vaccines come in two versions – inactivated, given by injection, or live attenuated (weakened), which are given by mouth (oral). In many countries, the oral vaccine is the only one available. Adults and older children need two doses, one to six weeks apart; younger children need three doses. The only people that need to be vaccinated are those who are going to come in close contact with cases, such as emergency relief workers or people working in laboratories handling the bacterium.

COVID-19

The undisputed heavyweight champion of the world (for now), COVID-19 is caused by a coronavirus. The coronavirus family are an evil lot. As well as being one of the causes of the common cold, the epidemics of SARS and MERS were caused by coronaviruses. They cause diarrhoea in pigs and cows and hepatitis and encephalitis in mice. The name is derived from the Latin word for crown. Very apt.

No-one knows for sure the origin of the COVID-19 virus, but it is now well and truly established in the human race, and will likely be with us for a long time to come, as it continues to mutate and find ways of escaping our immune systems.

COVID-19, like flu, is spread by sneezing, coughing and touching contaminated skin and other surfaces. The incubation period is two to twelve days; however, most cases of the original strain had an incubation period of around five or six days; this is shorter for the newer strains (three days for Omicron). Everyone knows the classic symptoms of a continuous cough, fever and change of taste or smell, but COVID-19 can cause a whole host of other symptoms, including breathlessness, muscle aches, headache, sore throat, diarrhoea and vomiting. The symptoms of the newer strains may be less typical, especially in people who have been vaccinated. Some people experience persistent symptoms, long COVID, with tiredness, shortness of breath, palpitations, dizziness, pins and needles, difficulty in concentrating, depression and disturbed sleep.

At the time of writing, there are currently thirty-eight different COVID-19 vaccines on the market, and nearly 200 waiting in the wings, in clinical trials. There are five types of approved vaccines: mRNA, viral vector, DNA, inactivated and protein subunit.

Most of the vaccines require two doses for full protection, although one (Johnson & Johnson) was effective after one dose in the original Phase 3 trial. With the emergence of variants, it is now clear that two doses plus two boosters are needed for optimum protection. At the time of writing, it is not clear how many additional boosters will be required, and when, although this seems likely, at least for people at risk of severe COVID-19. Vaccines are being adapted for new variants, and also for potential combination with influenza vaccine. The effectiveness of the current vaccines is greatest against hospitalisations and deaths, less so for mild disease. Vaccines also reduce your risk of catching the infection and transmitting it to other people.

Dengue Fever

This is a thoroughly modern disease. Although the first record of a case is in a Chinese medical encyclopaedia from the Jin Dynasty (265–420 AD), it only became a major problem following the rapid increase in travel and urbanisation that took place after World War II. The virus that causes dengue fever is spread by the bite of the *Aedes* species of mosquito, which lives in stagnant water, and causes epidemics in tropical and subtropical countries all over the world. I had dengue fever when I lived in St Lucia. I had a high fever and a rash, but the worst bit was the muscle pain. I felt like someone had set about me with a baseball bat. The pain of dengue is so severe that it's known as breakbone fever. In more severe cases, there is internal bleeding which is often fatal.

A live attenuated dengue vaccine was developed recently, and is available in some countries where the disease is common. It is only suitable for people who have already had the disease. This might sound like getting the vaccine is a waste of time, however, there are four strains of dengue virus, and as you only become immune to the one that infected you, the vaccine stops you from becoming reinfected with a different strain. The vaccine is given in three doses, six months apart.

Diphtheria

The reason I became involved in vaccines (Chapter 1). By coincidence, my father wrote his MD thesis on diphtheria. He died when I was four and I only discovered his thesis nearly fifty years later when clearing my mother's house after she died. By then, I had been working on vaccines for almost twenty years, so it was rather poignant to realise we shared the same passion.

Diphtheria is a respiratory infection, caused by a bacterium, *Corynebacterium diphtheriae*. It has a cousin called *Corynebacterium ulcerans* that sometimes contaminates unpasteurised milk. Diphtheria causes massive swelling of the throat and the soft tissues of the neck, making you look rather like a bull and obstructing breathing. The bacterium produces an incredibly powerful toxin that gets into your bloodstream and attacks the heart and nervous system. The fatal dose of diphtheria toxin for a seventy-kilogram adult is just seven micrograms – one-quarter of a millionth of an ounce. Just for the record, the most lethal toxin on the planet is botulinum toxin, fifty times more powerful than diphtheria toxin. Worth thinking about when you go for your next Botox injection.

The vaccine is made by inactivating the toxin to produce a toxoid. It works in two ways – by neutralising the effect of the toxin, and preventing people from carrying the disease. It is one of the basic childhood vaccines, given in various combinations with other antigens-tetanus, whooping cough, polio, hepatitis B and *Haemophilus influenzae* type b. There is a lower dose version for older children and adults, which also comes in combinations with tetanus, whooping cough and polio. The vaccine schedule is three doses, one to two months apart, with two boosters given before or during school.

Ebola

A very new kid on the block and a harbinger of things to come. Images of health workers in gowns and masks and mass burials flashed across our screens in 2014, as an epidemic ripped through West Africa. The epidemic killed over 11,000 people, many of them health workers, in Guinea, Liberia and Sierra Leone. Ebola is a member of another elite group of deadly pathogens, called viral haemorrhagic fevers, which include Yellow fever, Lassa fever and Marburg disease. Their victims literally bleed to death; only one in two people with Ebola will survive.

Ebola fever is spread between humans by infected blood and body fluids. No-one knows for sure where it first came from; the most likely theory is that it is carried by fruit bats who infect chimps, monkeys and other wild animals, jumping to humans by the eating of "bushmeat". The name comes from the Ebola River in the Democratic Republic of Congo, where one of the first outbreaks was discovered.

The World Health Organization declared the West African epidemic a public health emergency, and within a few months a large Phase 3 trial of a vaccine was underway in Guinea. The vaccine – which is a genetically engineered viral vector vaccine, was effective, and is now licensed and ready to be used again. The accelerated development paved the way for COVID-19; several of the vaccines now being used are made with the same technology as the Ebola vaccine.

Hib (*Haemophilus influenzae* type b)

Hib is a serious disease that affects young children, causing meningitis, septicaemia (blood poisoning) and sometimes epiglottitis (inflammation of the flap at the back of your tongue that stops food going down your windpipe). The disease is spread between children by coughing and sneezing. One in twenty children will die, and one in three are left with permanent complications of the nervous system – deafness, convulsions and mental impairment. *Haemophilus influenzae* is a bacterium that comes in six types, a–f, depending on the composition of the coat that covers its surface, called the capsule. Before vaccines came along most infections were due to the type b strain, so vaccines were developed for just that type. Vaccination has virtually eliminated the type b strain, so the only cases that are left are due to the other strains, or infections due to strains that don't have a capsule.

Hib vaccines belong to the group known as protein-polysaccharide conjugates. These vaccines are made by taking the outer capsule of the bacterium and linking it to a protein to improve the immune response. Vaccines for pneumococcal disease, some types of meningococcal meningitis and typhoid are made using the same technology. Hib is part of the routine childhood schedule, given to all babies in combination with other antigens as a three-dose schedule with a booster in the second year of life.

Hepatitis A

One of the less pleasant aspects of planning an exotic holiday used to be getting your hepatitis A immune globulin injection. This involved having a large volume of thick liquid (up to ten ml depending on your weight) injected into your buttock. It felt like a kick from a mule. Worse still, the protection only lasted a couple of months, so it had to be repeated every time you travelled. Our bottoms all heaved a collective sigh of relief when a vaccine that provided long-lasting protection came along in the 1990s.

Hepatitis A is a caused by a virus, with the rather unimaginative name of *Hepatovirus A*. A classic disease of poor hygiene, it is very common in countries with inadequate sanitation and poverty. As hygiene improves, the incidence of hepatitis A drops, making the disease a pretty good barometer of the cleanliness of a country. In developed countries, it mainly affects homeless people, injecting drug users and men who have sex with men. Uncooked or lightly cooked shellfish are also risky as they are filter feeders, building up huge concentrations of the virus if they are grown in sewage-contaminated water. I have a particular penchant for raw oysters with a twist of lemon and shallots. Hurrah for the vaccine.

Hepatitis A attacks your liver, turning you yellow (jaundice) with nausea, diarrhoea and vomiting. About one percent of people will die from liver failure. Definitely worth avoiding. The vaccine is made from an inactivated live virus. Two doses six months apart will give you long-term protection, but one dose will protect you short term as long as you have the vaccine at least two weeks before you travel. Sometimes it is combined with other travel vaccines such as typhoid and hepatitis B. In the United States and a couple of other countries, the vaccine is given to all children to prevent the spread of the disease in nurseries.

Hepatitis B

Hepatitis A's rather more unpleasant sibling. This is a blood-borne virus that stalks us via blood transfusions, shared drug injection needles, tattooing, ear piercing, acupuncture and unprotected sex, to name a few. What makes this villain so unpleasant is that about one in ten people who catch it become long-term carriers. The virus persists in your blood and slowly starts killing your liver cells, turning it into a lump of leather-like scar tissue, better known as cirrhosis. If you're really unlucky, the cells become cancerous. The WHO estimates there are 250 million carriers of hepatitis B in the world, and nearly 1 million people die every year from related cirrhosis and liver cancer. Once you're a carrier, you're a carrier for life and can infect other people. This is particularly dangerous in pregnancy – a baby born to a mother carrying the virus starts life with a ninety percent chance of becoming a lifelong carrier.

The virus that causes hepatitis B was discovered in 1965 by Baruch Blumberg, an American physician and geneticist. He first isolated it from an indigenous Australian; the virus was initially known as the Australia antigen. Blumberg's work earned him the Nobel prize and paved the way for vaccines. The hepatitis B vaccine in use today was the first vaccine to be produced using gene-based technology. It is given to all babies as part of the combination of other antigens. Three doses are enough for lifelong protection. The vaccine is also available on its own for adults that didn't get the vaccine as a child. It's recommended for people who are at risk, such as healthcare workers, injecting drug users and people who need regular transfusions. There is also a version combined with hepatitis A, which is handy for travellers.

Hepatitis E

You may ask what happened to hepatitis C and D? The hepatitis viruses are named in the order they were discovered. C and D do exist, but there are no vaccines, although it would be jolly handy if there were, especially for hepatitis C, which is another blood-borne infection that can persist and lead to cirrhosis and cancer. There are several hepatitis C vaccines in development. Hepatitis D, better known as delta hepatitis, is a virus that only infects people who already have hepatitis B, a double whammy, making it even more likely that you will experience complications. If you are vaccinated against hepatitis B, you cannot develop delta hepatitis.

Hepatitis E is more like hepatitis A, spread by contaminated food and water. It is particularly common in Asia, but appears to be on the increase in Europe. It gets a mention here because there is a vaccine, although at the moment it is only used in China.

Human Papillomavirus (HPV)

HPV has the rather dubious distinction of being the virus that causes cancer of the cervix, the fourth most common cancer in the world. The virus is spread during sex and most people will be infected at some point in their life. There are at least 170 types of HPV, most of which are harmless, however, a handful have the ability to persist and slowly change the cells in the cervix to become pre-cancerous, then cancerous, over many years. These types can also cause cancer of the anus, penis, vagina, head and neck. Other HPV types cause genital warts. Few viruses have the ability to cause so many different diseases.

The vaccine is made from bits of the outer coat of the virus, known as virus-like particles, VLPs. These VLPs are genetically engineered, grown in either yeast cells or cells derived from a type of moth. Because it only contains parts of the virus, it is not living, so can't replicate. The latest version of the vaccine contains nine of the most common types; seven that cause cancer and two that cause genital warts. Earlier versions contained two or four types.

The vaccine is given to young adolescents, who (hopefully) have not started having sex. Initially, it was only given to girls, but more and more countries have started vaccinating boys. Two or three doses are needed. It takes many years to see the impact on cervical cancer, but in November 2021, a paper published in the Lancet showed that cervical cancer cases had been cut by nearly ninety percent in the UK. The UK started using the vaccine in 2008. HPV has the potential to be the first ever vaccine to eliminate a cancer. One thing less for my three daughters to worry about.

Influenza

A disease that needs no introduction, influenza is one of the "big five" pandemic diseases. It caused the famous Spanish flu pandemic of 1918–1920, which killed as many as 50 million people. The name Spanish flu has nothing to do with where the pandemic started (this is still unknown). Spain had remained neutral during World War I, so there was no censoring of the press. In the United States and the rest of Europe, governments suppressed bad stories that might affect morale. The Spanish press reported the pandemic in full gory detail, including the illness of the king, Alfonso XIII, who nearly died from the infection. This gave the distorted impression that the pandemic was much worse in Spain, giving it the name (it was also called Spanish Lady). Other countries called it different names based on where they thought it originated: In Senegal it was named the "Brazilian flu", and in Brazil the "German flu" while in Poland it was known as the "Bolshevik disease". There have been smaller flu pandemics in 1957, 1968, 1977 and 2009, but nothing on the same scale as the 1918– 1920 pandemic.

Many people use the word flu to describe mild respiratory illnesses, but the real thing is very unpleasant. My mother and I both had flu during the 1957 pandemic. We were poleaxed for a fortnight and felt exhausted for several weeks.

The problem with the flu virus is that it is continually mutating. Usually, these changes are small, but sometimes there is a significant change that throws up a new strain that no-one is immune to. An average of 650,000 people die from flu around the world every year, but when a new strain appears, the figure can be much higher (but still nowhere near the toll from COVID-19, which has already claimed over 6 million lives). Older people and people with conditions like chronic bronchitis, diabetes, kidney failure and liver cirrhosis (hardening of the liver) are particularly at risk.

Flu vaccine manufacture is a bit of a nightmare. The World Health Organization tracks the evolution of the virus around the world, and every year tells manufacturers which strains to include in the vaccine. Then it's a race against time to produce the new vaccine before the flu season starts. By the time the vaccines are produced, the strains causing the most disease may be different. The strain match is better in some years than others. The other problem is that most flu vaccines are made using eggs. The virus is grown on fertilised chicken eggs; these are highly specialised eggs that have been certified as safe for vaccine production. This is a major bottleneck in the supply. Each dose of flu vaccine needs three or four eggs. That's an awful lot of hens. Currently, all the world's flu manufacturers together are not able to produce enough vaccine to vaccinate everyone. Some vaccines can now be produced without relying on eggs.

Most of the vaccines are inactivated; there is one live attenuated vaccine that is given by nasal spray.

The vaccine has to be given every year. The recommendations for flu vaccine have expanded recently. Initially, it was recommended just for the elderly and people with chronic illnesses. Nowadays, many countries also recommend the vaccine for children and pregnant women. Healthcare workers are also a priority for the vaccine, although this is mainly to stop them spreading the disease to their patients. Most vaccines today contain four strains of the virus: two A strains and two B strains.

Japanese Encephalitis

Another exotic disease, also rather unfairly named after one country, as it occurs throughout Asia. It is caused by a virus which is carried by pigs; it gets to humans via the bite of a mosquito that likes to live in paddy fields. Most people have no symptoms, or very mild ones, but occasionally there is inflammation of the brain, encephalitis, which can cause all kinds of unpleasant symptoms including a splitting headache, confusion and convulsions. About half of people who develop encephalitis are left with permanent brain damage.

The vaccine is a killed viral vaccine; the schedule is two doses a month apart. It's a traveller's vaccine, but you only need it if you are planning to spend long periods of time in the Asian countryside, where there is pig farming and rice growing.

Leptospirosis

The next time you go open water swimming, it would be a jolly good idea to make sure you have covered any cuts with plasters, and have a long shower afterwards. The water might be contaminated with the urine of rats and other animals, and they carry a very unpleasant bacterial infection: leptospirosis. This is a thankfully rare occupational hazard for farmers and sewage workers, and a recreational hazard of outdoor water sports.

The disease is named after the genus of the *Leptospira* bacteria. The early symptoms are fever, headache, muscle ache and eye redness. This subsides, but sometimes there is a second phase, with meningitis and inflammation of the kidneys, liver and other organs. In the most severe cases – called Weil's disease – there is jaundice and kidney failure, which can be fatal.

There is a killed vaccine, but it has limited effectiveness as it only protects against one of the many strains that cause the illness. It is only available in a few countries (France is one) where it is recommended for people at high risk of being exposed. The schedule is two doses a fortnight apart, with a booster at six months and further boosters every ten years if you are at continuing risk. There is a version of the vaccine for dogs, who like nothing more than rolling around in rat infested ditches. My dog Jack, a lively terrier, gets his leptospirosis jab every year.

Malaria

One the greatest infectious disease scourges remaining on the planet, along with TB, HIV and now COVID-19. A third of the world's population lives in countries affected by malaria. It kills 400,000 people a year; half of them in Africa. Malaria is an ancient disease; remnants of the parasite have been found in fossilised tree resin dating back 30 million years. It has probably had more impact on society than any other infectious disease. At some point in its history, malaria has been present in every continent, apart from Antarctica. It has shaped the course of history, striking down monarchs, popes and military leaders. Otto II, King of the Germans and Emperor of Rome, died from malaria in 983. Alexander the Great is believed to have died from malaria in 232 BC, on route to India. So many popes died of malaria that in the fourteenth century, foreign popes were not allowed to live in Rome due to fear of "Roman Fever". The name "malaria" means "bad air" in mediaeval Italian (it was believed to come from pestilential fumes in swamps). During the American Civil War of 1861–1865, it was estimated that fifty percent of white soldiers and eighty percent of black soldiers got malaria annually. In World War II, 60,000 US troops died from malaria. In 1943, General Douglas MacArthur said: "This will be a long war if for every division I have facing the enemy I must count on a second division in hospital with malaria and a third division convalescing from this debilitating disease."

The cause is neither a bacterium nor a virus, but a single-celled microorganism called *Plasmodium*. There are various species, of which one, *Plasmodium falciparum*, is particularly deadly. Humans become infected by blood-sucking mosquitos. The *Plasmodium* travels to the liver, then red blood cells, metamorphosing into different forms on its journey. Malaria can produce almost any symptom, but the classic one is a sudden high fever with rigor, an uncontrollable shaking. More serious cases affect the brain (cerebral malaria), liver (bilious malaria), heart and lungs (algid malaria), and many other organs.

I've included malaria because a vaccine has been approved and is currently being rolled out in sub-Saharan Africa. It's a complex construct, with genetically engineered proteins derived from the *Plasmodium*, hepatitis B antigen, which improves the immune response, and an adjuvant. It has taken more than twenty years of painstaking research to develop the world's first malaria vaccine, and more are in the pipeline.

Measles

If there was an award for the most tenacious infectious disease, measles would win hands down. Vaccination had almost eliminated measles from the developed world by the end of the twentieth century; it is now the comeback kid of the twenty first. The epidemic of measles that flared up in Europe in 2017 has affected every country, claiming nearly a hundred lives.

David Salisbury, who was head of the UK Immunisation Programme, said that tracking measles is like watching car windscreen wipers. You see the rain, then it's gone, then it's back, then it's gone; on and on. Measles owes its ability to cause epidemics to its infectiousness. The R_0, the basic reproduction number, can be as high as eighteen, depending on the setting. Imagine every case of measles giving it to eighteen people, and each of those eighteen people giving it to eighteen more and so on. You don't need to be good at maths to see that you very quickly get to an epidemic. The next most infectious disease is chickenpox, with an R_0 of a mere twelve.

Measles is caused by a virus that belongs to the *Morbillivirus* group. These viruses affect humans and animals. They cause distemper in dogs, with cough, fever, diarrhoea and thickening of the footpads and rinderpest, a severe infection with fever and diarrhoea that affects sheep, goats, cattle and other hooved animals. I'm always amazed how such closely related viruses can cause completely different illnesses between animals and humans. Measles is spread by respiratory droplets and direct contact with secretions from the nose and throat, another good reason why it moves so fast between younger citizens. A snotty-nosed toddler with measles can infect an entire nursery, doctor's waiting room or birthday party within minutes. Measles often develops into all kinds of complications, including ear infections, pneumonia, convulsions and encephalitis. The author Roald Dahl's daughter, Olivia, died aged seven from measles encephalitis in 1962, a year before the vaccine became available. Sometimes the virus persists in the brain, causing subacute sclerosing panencephalitis, SSPE. This is a slow, progressive neurological condition that comes on several years after the acute illness. It starts with behaviour changes, then intellectual deterioration, convulsions and blindness. It's always fatal and there is no cure.

Measles vaccine is a live attenuated vaccine. Nowadays, it's usually given in combination with mumps and rubella, MMR. Some combinations also include the chickenpox vaccine. Children get the vaccine after their first birthday and a second dose a few years later (anywhere between two and thirteen years old, depending on the country), to make sure they have long-term protection. Because the vaccine is live, it can't be given to children with weakened immune systems, for example those being treated for leukaemia.

Meningococcal Disease

Measles may win the prize for the most infectious disease, but meningococcal disease is definitely a contender for the most frightening. The bacterium, *Neisseria meningitidis*, can overwhelm your defences in a few hours, getting into the bloodstream and affecting every organ in your body. I have only seen one case, a teenage girl who needed an amputation to stop its spread. It's every doctor's nightmare.

The disease is often referred to as meningitis, which is a bit misleading. Meningitis is inflammation of the meninges, the membranes that surround your brain and spinal cord, cushioning them against injury. *Neisseria meningitidis* can certainly cause meningitis, but so can lots of other bacteria, several viruses and even some protozoa. While meningitis is extremely unpleasant (the headache is unbearable) the worst consequences of meningococcal disease are when the bacterium gets into your blood stream; this is bacteraemia, also called septicaemia. The bacterium becomes rampant, shutting down your vital organs. One in ten people will die. If you are lucky enough to survive, you have a one in seven chance of being left with permanent deafness, convulsions, loss of intellect or an amputation.

The disease is spread, like other respiratory infections, via droplets and direct contact with nose and throat secretions. Roughly one in ten people carry the bacterium harmlessly in the nose and throat. The reason why some people get the disease rather than become carriers isn't really understood. Smoking seems to be a factor and so does crowding, hence the outbreaks in army barracks, university campuses and the annual Haj pilgrimage to Mecca.

Another problem with this disease is that the only way to get a certain diagnosis is with a lab test. Other causes of bacterial meningitis can cause the same symptoms so you need a sample of blood or cerebrospinal fluid (the liquid that lubricates your meninges) to identify the culprit.

There are thirteen different strains (known as serogroups) of *Neisseria meningitidis*, but six of them cause disease: A, B, C, W-135, X and Y. Serogroups, B, C and Y are the most common worldwide, although W is increasing in some countries.

There are vaccines for all the disease-causing strains except X. Vaccines for serogroups A, C, W-135 and Y are protein-polysaccharide conjugates, made using the same technology as for Hib and pneumococcal vaccines, linking the outer capsule of the bacterium to a protein, to give a strong, lasting immune response. The vaccine either has all four serogroups in one combination, or just one on its own, either A or C. There is also a version where a serogroup C vaccine is combined with Hib. Serogroup B vaccines are made from genetically engineered proteins, and currently only exist as versions on their own, although combinations are under development.

The schedules for meningococcal vaccines vary for the different types of vaccines and the recommendations of the country. Meningococcal B vaccines are either given to babies (three doses) or to teenagers and sometimes young adults (two doses). Vaccines for A, C, W and Y are usually given to children at around one year (sometimes older), with a second dose in their teens.

Mumps

Press your finger into your cheek, between the bottom of your ear and your jawbone. You should feel something squidgy with a bumpy surface. This is your parotid gland, and it's important for two reasons: it keeps your mouth topped up with saliva, and is also the organ that swells up when you get mumps. Mumps is another disease spread by respiratory droplets. People think of mumps as unpleasant, but not serious. In fact, the mumps virus, which rejoices in the name *Orthorubulavirus*, can attack the pancreas, ovaries, testes (yes guys, it's painful), meninges, kidneys, joint and heart. It's particularly unpleasant if you get it as an adult. Sara, my oldest daughter, caught mumps in her final year at university. She had been vaccinated many years before, but at that time no booster was given (this changed later). It knocked her for six; she looked like a hamster, was exhausted, and couldn't concentrate properly for several weeks. She got her degree, but it was a struggle.

Mumps is a live attenuated vaccine. It is given as part of the MMR vaccine, in a two-dose schedule.

Plague

Strictly speaking, this disease shouldn't appear in my line up of villains, as the vaccine was discontinued a few years ago (new improved ones are being developed). However, I couldn't resist a few words on the disease that has caused the greatest pandemic of all time – the Black Death. In the fourteenth century, Genoese merchant ships carried their goods from Asia to the

Middle East, Africa and Europe. They also carried millions of black rats, infected with *Yersinia pestis*, the bacterium that causes plague. The disease spread to humans via fleas, who would feed on the rats, becoming infected themselves. A flea with plague is hungry and humans made a tasty alternative to rats. An infected flea would bite an unsuspecting sailor, then thoughtfully proceed to vomit infected blood into the wound. The fourteenth century plague pandemic killed up to 200 million people in seven years, more than a third of the world's population. COVID-19 pales in significance compared to the impact this had on society; it took two centuries for the population of Europe to recover.

Plague comes in two forms: bubonic plague, affecting the lymphatic system (bubo is the word to describe a swollen lymph node) and pneumonic plague, affecting the lungs. The well-known children's nursery rhyme is thought to be about plague: Ring-a-ring o' roses (red blotches on the skin), a pocket full of posies (people carried sweet-smelling flowers to ward off plague), a-tishoo! a-tishoo! (sneezing fits in pneumonic plague), we all fall down (dying).

Humans with pneumonic plague are infectious to other humans, which is why the disease spread so rapidly from the merchant ships. In an effort to control plague, the Port of Venice made ships stay offshore for forty days before discharging their goods, giving us the word quarantine (*quarante* is Italian for forty). Sailors who had the plague died on board and were tipped over the side, where they were no longer a public health problem.

Plague has caused many pandemics over the centuries, but none greater than the Black Death. It is still present today in a few countries, including the United States, where the occasional hapless tourist in Yosemite National Park is bitten by a plague-infected flea.

Pneumococcal Disease

A somewhat lesser-known character, the bacterium *Streptococcus pneumoniae* is nevertheless a colourful customer, existing as more than a hundred different strains. Like meningococcal disease, many people are carriers, and being a carrier makes you immune to the strain you are carrying.

Pneumococcal disease affects people at the extremes of life. In the elderly it causes pneumonia; young children get pneumonia but also meningitis, ear infections and bacteraemia (blood poisoning, also known as septicaemia).

There are two main types of pneumococcal vaccines. The vaccine given to children is another protein-polysaccharide conjugate, like Hib and meningococcal A, C, W and Y vaccines. It is given to babies, with two or three doses. The vaccine contains the strains that cause the most disease; either ten or thirteen strains depending on the manufacturer. The vaccine usually given to older people is a plain polysaccharide. It is made from the outer capsule of the bacterium, but there is no added protein. It contains the twenty-three most common strain-strains. Conjugate vaccines containing fifteen or twenty strains have recently been approved and are now recommended for adults in the United States.

Polio

Anyone who grew up in the late 1940s and early 1950s will remember the terror of polio epidemics. The disease paralyses your muscles, often leaving you permanently disabled. In the most severe version, it attacks your diaphragm, stopping you from being able to expand your chest and take a breath. Thousands of polio victims spent their lives in an iron lung. The epidemics were indiscriminate. Famous polio survivors include the actress Mia Farrow, golfer Jack Nicklaus and Ian Dury of the Blockheads. The most famous polio survivor, Franklin D Roosevelt, probably had Guillain–Barré syndrome, not polio.

Although it attacks the nervous system, polio is actually a gut infection. People with polio excrete the virus, which can survive for weeks in sewage, soil and water. Paradoxically, the post-war epidemics were actually a consequence of improved living standards. In the first half of the twentieth century, when hygiene was poor, everyone caught polio as a child. Polio in a child is usually a mild illness, or causes no symptoms at all. As living conditions improved, people didn't catch the disease until they were older. Polio in an adult is a very different ballgame; one in ten people infected will develop paralysis, usually with some permanent disability. As the disease shifted from children to adults, cases of paralysis became more and more common.

Polio has now all but been eradicated by vaccination. There are two versions of the vaccine – live attenuated and killed. The live attenuated version is given by mouth. Obviously, this is a huge advantage, especially during mass campaigns, however, it does have one drawback: the vaccine can occasionally change back to a more virulent form and cause paralysis. In an attempt to work out exactly how this happens, I once got hold of the contents of several hundred nappies of recently vaccinated babies (don't ask me how) and invited Philip Minor, a virologist with a large laboratory, stamina and a good sense of humour, to analyse them. He diligently looked for poliovirus in every poo of thirty babies for a month after getting vaccinated. He found multiple mutations in the virus, particularly of one type (there are three strains), and some of the babies excreted the virus for the entire month following vaccination. Another reason to wash your hands after changing a nappy.

The other type of polio vaccine is a killed vaccine and is the most commonly used version nowadays. It doesn't cause paralysis, but has to be given by injection. It's usually given in combination with the other childhood routine vaccines.

A full course of polio vaccine is three doses as a baby, with two boosters later in childhood.

Q Fever

A disease with an unusual name caused by an unusual bacterium. *Coxiella burnetii* is another organism that can form hardy spores that survive heat, drying and chemicals. Once it infects its prey, however, the bacterium can only survive inside its host's cells, rather like a virus. Q fever is transmitted to humans mainly from sheep, goats and cattle, by inhaling the spores or touching surfaces that they have contaminated. Animals with Q fever are particularly infectious during childbirth.

The symptoms of Q fever are headache, fever, muscle ache and cough, but it can also affect lungs, liver, heart and the nervous system. Some people develop chronic fatigue which can last for years.

There is an inactivated vaccine, which is currently only available in Australia. It is given as a single dose, with no boosters. It is only recommended for people who have close animal contact, like vets and farmers.

Rabies

This is a real Hammer Horror disease. Someone with rabies has violent jerky movements, progressive paralysis, extreme anxiety, confusion, and sometimes the classical symptom of hydrophobia, becoming terrified at the sight of water. Virtually everyone dies, slowly, over weeks and sometimes months.

Rabies is a viral infection, caused by a *Lyssavirus*. Most people get rabies from a dog bite, but many other animals can transmit the disease, including bats, skunks, raccoons and foxes. Luckily it is relatively rare. Vaccination of wild and domestic animals has almost eliminated the disease in Europe, and most human cases occur in Africa and Asia. There is a killed viral vaccine that is recommended for people going to high-risk countries, particularly if they are likely to be bitten by a dog (cycling, hiking or feeding a cute stray dog are all invitations to get bitten). It is a course of three injections over a month. If you are unlucky enough to get bitten in a high-risk country, an immunoglobulin can also be given, in an effort to give you some immunity to fight off the disease while the vaccine response kicks in.

Rotavirus

This is a highly democratic virus. Virtually every child will get infected at least once by the time they celebrate their fifth birthday. It causes diarrhoea, which is usually short-lived, however, babies become dehydrated very easily, so sometimes they end up in hospital. In developed countries, babies usually recover quickly, but it's a very different story in less well-off countries. Severe dehydration from rotavirus is often fatal, with half a million children dying every year.

Rotavirus spreads very easily between young children. Good hygiene helps control spread, but isn't enough. Before vaccines came along, there was an epidemic every winter, like clockwork. As many as a third of the beds in children's hospital wards were occupied by rotavirus patients.

The vaccine is live, attenuated and given by mouth. Babies get either two or three doses, depending on the manufacturer. It's a live vaccine, so it can't be given to babies with severely suppressed immune systems (this is a very small number of babies). Very rarely the vaccine causes a condition known as intussusception. This is a when a bit of the bowel folds in on itself, causing a blockage. It often resolves on its own, but sometimes requires surgery. In countries that have introduced the vaccine, hospital admissions for diarrhoea in babies have plummeted; interrupting transmission of the virus has also reduced the disease in older children, who didn't get the vaccine. Herd immunity at work.

Rubella

Better known as German measles (it used to be considered as a variant of measles until a German doctor described it as a separate disease), this is the virus that pregnant women used to dread. If you were infected in the first two months of pregnancy you had a ninety percent chance of giving birth to a baby with multiple defects. Babies with congenital rubella syndrome usually have mental disability, are often deaf, with cataracts and heart defects. In one epidemic in the United States, 20,000 babies were born with congenital rubella syndrome. Many women opted to terminate the pregnancy if they found out they had been infected.

Rubella is a viral infection, caused by the *Rubivirus*. It looks a bit like measles, with fever and a rash, and is spread in the same way, by respiratory droplets. Adults sometimes get inflamed joints.

The arrival of a live attenuated vaccine in 1969 was a godsend. We have to thank two of the giants of the vaccine world: Maurice Hilleman who first developed it, and Stanley Plotkin, who improved it. It is given as part of the MMR vaccine, in a two-dose schedule.

Shingles

Inside your nerve cells, a virus is sleeping. It has been there for decades. Then it wakes up, and all hell breaks loose. At first, it's just a tingling sensation, but soon, blisters erupt on your skin and the tingling becomes a searing pain. If you're lucky, it goes after a couple of weeks. Many are not so lucky. The rash goes but the pain doesn't. In a condition called postherpetic neuralgia, the pain can last for months after the rash has healed. Some people can't even bear the touch of clothing on the skin. The virus can also spread to your lungs, liver, heart, gut and brain. You can die. Shingles is no picnic.

The virus that causes shingles, *varicella-zoster* virus, is the same one that causes chickenpox. It becomes dormant (the medical term is latent) in your nerve cells, and is reactivated many years later, as your immune system starts to age. Diseases that suppress your immune system like HIV, and some cancers, can also lead to reactivation. The reactivated virus affects one or more nerves, and the painful rash appears on the areas of skin supplied by that nerve. A particularly nasty version affects the nerve that supplies your eye, causing loss of vision. Someone with shingles can transmit the virus to another person, giving them chickenpox, but you can't catch shingles from someone who has chickenpox.

There are two types of shingles vaccine, a live attenuated one and a genetically engineered version that contains a bit of protein from the virus and an adjuvant. The live version needs just one dose; the protein-adjuvant version needs two doses given two to six months apart. Shingles vaccination is recommended for older people; the age depends on the country and which vaccine is available. In the United States, it is recommended for everybody above fifty, using the two-dose vaccine. In the UK, where both vaccines are currently available, the age cut-off is seventy. The UK chose a higher cut-off age because the disease is most severe in the elderly, and it is more cost-effective to concentrate on vaccinating this age group.

Smallpox

Although the WHO declared the world free from smallpox in 1980, there are still stocks of the virus in two laboratories, one in Russia and one in the United States. The main argument for not destroying these last remnants of the virus is the threat of biological warfare. There are various types of vaccines, made from a virus called *Vaccinia* which is related to the *Variola* virus that causes smallpox, but is harmless. The vaccine used for the WHO smallpox eradication campaign was given using a two-pronged needle which is dipped into the vaccine then used to prick the skin several times. A few days later, a sore develops which blisters, then forms a scab which falls off leaving a scar. According to my childhood vaccination booklet (yes, I still have it, sad person that I am), I have had smallpox vaccine five times. I can only find one scar though (on the side of my calf of all places). Now the disease has been eradicated, no-one gets vaccinated, apart from a few laboratory workers who continue to work with viruses that are closely related to smallpox, such as monkeypox. Despite its name, monkeypox occurs mainly in rodents, and occasionally infects humans in parts of Africa.

Tetanus

Tetanus, like diphtheria, is a disease caused by the toxin that the bacterium produces. The culprit is *Clostridium tetani* that lives, in a dormant state, in soil and manure. When you stand on a dirty nail or garden fork, the bacterium gets under your skin and wakes up. About ten days later, muscle stiffness sets in. The first muscles affected are often those that move your jaw, hence the name lockjaw. The stiffness soon turns into painful, spasmodic contractions, affecting muscles of the chest, neck, back and abdomen. The contractions can be so violent that you break bones and shatter muscles. Contracted back muscles arch you backwards, turning you into a circus acrobat. The diaphragm can be affected, making you struggle for every breath. Even with the best intensive care treatment, about ten percent of people with tetanus die. A particularly nasty version occurs in newborn babies, who get infected through the umbilical stump that has been cut with a non-sterile instrument. It occurs mainly in developing countries. Vaccination of pregnant women and improved hygiene during delivery has greatly reduced the incidence in recent years.

Tetanus vaccine is a toxoid, made by killing the toxin. It is given in combination with other childhood vaccines as a course of three doses in infancy with two boosters later in childhood. Booster doses are sometimes needed when you have an injury that is prone to tetanus.

Tick-Borne Encephalitis

One of the lesser-known vaccine-preventable diseases, this is a viral infection that occurs in parts of central and eastern Europe, Scandinavia, the Baltics, the former Soviet Republics and China. It used to be particularly common in Austria (everyone there gets vaccinated now), where it rejoices in the name of Frühsommer-Meningoenzephalitis, or early summer meningo-encephalitis.

Humans get the disease from a tick, which lives in forests and feeds on all kinds of rodents, birds, dogs, sheep and goats. It's usually a mild flu-like illness, but sometimes it progresses, affecting the meninges and brain.

There is a killed vaccine, given as three doses over six to twelve months. You only need the vaccine if you are planning on hiking or camping in affected areas.

Tuberculosis

There is a well-known graph that shows the incidence of tuberculosis in the UK from the start of the twentieth century to the present day. The line moves steadily downwards throughout the twentieth century. The discovery of the first antibiotic to treat tuberculosis, streptomycin, has little effect on the rate of decline, nor does the introduction of BCG vaccine in 1953. You might be tempted to think that neither of these interventions had any impact and that the disease was disappearing on its own. What the graph is actually showing is that tuberculosis is a disease that is directly linked to living standards. As conditions improved steadily, cases dropped. Then, at the start of the twenty-first century, the decline abruptly stops. Cases start to rise in some parts of the country, especially London. Homelessness, injecting drug use and rise of antibiotic resistance have all played a part. Tuberculosis is not going away any time soon.

The bacterium responsible is *Mycobacterium tuberculosis*. It is spread by coughing, sneezing or even singing and prolonged talking. The bacterium heads for the lungs, where one of three things happens. The body's immune system clears the infection; or the infection isn't cleared and becomes dormant (the technical term is latent) without causing symptoms; or you get full-blown tuberculosis. The classic symptoms are a cough with sputum which often has blood in it, fever, night sweats and weight loss. Tuberculosis can spread from the lungs to attack the meninges, bones, joints and lymph nodes. A quarter of the world's population has been infected, either as the latent or active form.

BCG is a live bacterial vaccine. The letters stand for Bacille Calmette–Guérin, named after the two French scientists who discovered it. It is best given at birth, but can also be given to older children and young adults. In this situation, a skin test needs to be done beforehand to check if you have already been infected, which rules out having the vaccine. The vaccine is a one-dose shot. An ulcer forms at the injection site, which heals up, often leaving a scar. This is rather useful, as it is an easy way to tell if someone has been vaccinated. As the vaccine is live, it can't be given to people with weakened immune systems.

Not all countries use BCG vaccine nowadays, particularly in Europe and North America. In others, for example the UK, it is given to people who are at higher risk, such as healthcare workers or babies living in inner cities, where the disease is still rife.

Typhoid

You are only likely to encounter typhoid fever, and its slightly less unpleasant cousin, paratyphoid fever, as a traveller. This is a disease of poor sanitation and hygiene, spread by contaminated food and water. It is particularly common in India and Pakistan. Typhoid fever is a bacterial infection caused by one of the members of the infamous food poisoning family, the *Salmonellae*. Typhoid is much more than a bout of food poisoning. Victims can suffer diarrhoea, fever, vomiting, constipation, abdominal pain, muscle aches, chills, headache, extreme tiredness, breathing difficulty, inflammation of the liver, spleen and other organs. Sometimes, people recover, but become long-term carriers, the most famous of whom was Mary Mallon, "Typhoid Mary", the itinerant Irish cook who managed to give typhoid to over fifty well-heeled New Yorkers between 1900 and 1915. She spent the rest of her life in quarantine.

There are two versions of the vaccine. One is made from the outside capsule of the bacterium, *Salmonella typhi*, and is given as a single injection. There is also a live attenuated version, which is given by mouth; the course is three doses, two days apart. Both vaccines will protect you for up to three years.

Varicella

Better known as chickenpox, the full-blown disease is unforgettable. Crops of blisters appear on the face, then the trunk, and finally the arms and legs. The blisters crust over, turning into scabs, only to be replaced by successive waves of new blisters. A child with chickenpox looks like something from a horror movie. As ghastly as it looks, most children recover quite quickly, with just a few scars as a reminder. For some people, however, chickenpox is a catastrophe. If you catch it when you're pregnant, it has all kinds of consequences. Chickenpox in early pregnancy can damage the growing fetus, in a condition known as congenital varicella syndrome, with missing limbs, a small head, cataracts and scarred skin. Mercifully, most such babies don't survive. Catching chickenpox later in pregnancy can give the newborn baby shingles. And if you catch chickenpox in the week just before or after giving birth, the result is a very severe attack of chickenpox for the baby, which can be fatal. People with weakened immune systems don't fare much better. The virus can attack the lungs, the liver, and cause widespread clotting of their blood vessels.

Chickenpox vaccine is a live attenuated viral vaccine. It can be given on its own, or in combination with the measles/mumps/rubella (MMR) vaccine. You need two doses for protection. Some countries give it to all children, in other countries it is only recommended for people at particular risk, for example a child who is about to start chemotherapy for cancer. There is also a specific immunoglobulin which can be given to provide immediate protection for someone who has been exposed to chickenpox and is at high risk of complications, such as a newborn baby.

Whooping Cough

In China, it's known as the Hundred Day Cough. That's how long, on average, a child will cough for. The victim endures repeated bouts of forceful coughing (doctors call them paroxysms), up to fifty a day. The whoop is the noise made by the sudden intake of air, the desperate gasp for breath that comes at the end of each paroxysm. Sometimes the whoop is replaced by a vomit. Oxygen starvation during a coughing fit literally turns you blue in the face. The coughing can be so intense and prolonged that blood vessels rupture, causing nosebleeds, bloodshot eyes and sometimes brain haemorrhages. Ribs are broken, hernias pop out. The child becomes dehydrated, loses weight and is completely exhausted. Pneumonia is a common complication. The lack of oxygen can cause permanent brain damage. Small babies fare particularly badly. They don't always have the typical symptoms, they splutter and choke, rather than whoop. Most deaths from whooping cough are in babies under three months of age, who are too young to have been vaccinated; whooping cough is one of the causes of sudden infant death.

This is a bacterial infection caused by *Bordetella pertussis* (hence its medical name, pertussis). The disease is transmitted by droplets during coughing fits, and is highly infectious (R_0 between five and six). The vaccine is a subunit vaccine, made from the components of the bacterium responsible for the symptoms of whooping cough. The components of these subunit vaccines protect against the effects of the disease but also help prevent you becoming infected. The vaccine is given to babies, in combination with the other childhood vaccines, with a booster injection before school. Some countries also offer the vaccine to pregnant women. This ensures that the newborn baby, who is at its most vulnerable, will be protected until old enough to be vaccinated themselves. The adult version of the vaccine also comes as a combination, with diphtheria, tetanus and polio antigens. As well as pregnant women, it can be given to any adult who didn't get the vaccine as a child, and some countries recommend a booster dose for all adults.

Yellow Fever

The ships that sailed from Africa to the New World in the seventeenth century carried more than slaves. On board was a mosquito called *Aedes aegypti*, carrying a deadly new disease. The first outbreak of Yellow fever in the Western Hemisphere occurred in Barbados, in 1647. From there it spread quickly to the rest of the Caribbean, then to North, Central and South America. An outbreak in Philadelphia in 1793 killed ten percent of the city and forced the government that was based there at the time to flee, including President George Washington. There were multiple outbreaks of Yellow fever in North and Central America, and the Caribbean, during the nineteenth century. It halted France's efforts to build the first Panama Canal.

The disease is caused by a virus from the flavivirus group. Flaviviruses are a nasty bunch, which also cause dengue, tick-borne encephalitis and Zika. It gets its name from the yellow appearance of the skin, due to jaundice. The initial symptoms are a bit like flu with fever, chills, nausea, headache and muscle aches. Some people recover, but many cases progress, with liver damage (hence the jaundice) and bleeding. Victims often vomit blood. Between twenty and thirty percent of people who develop jaundice will die. There is no cure.

The mosquito transmits the disease between humans and from monkeys to humans. Yellow fever is only found in Africa and Central and South America, but the *Aedes aegypti* mosquito exists in many other countries, especially Asia, which is why people travelling to some countries need a certificate to show they have been vaccinated. Travellers are vaccinated to stop the spread of the disease. It's a live attenuated vaccine and a single dose gives lifelong protection.

The Jargon

One of my pet hates is the medical jargon that doctors use to explain stuff to their patients. The world of vaccination is no different. Here is a list of the most commonly used terms and abbreviations. I've explained most of them throughout the book, they are listed together here for easy reference.

Terms

Adjuvant An additive that is used to strengthen the immune response to a vaccine. From the Latin word *adjuvare* (to help).

Adverse event Any medical condition that occurs after vaccination, but is not necessarily caused by it. The same term applies to medical conditions that occur after giving drugs.

Anaphylaxis A severe life-threatening allergic reaction that comes on very quickly after exposure to a foreign substance.

Antibody A protein that is produced by cells in your immune system which can combat viruses, bacteria and other microorganisms.

Antigen The part of the microorganism that is recognised by your immune system, and stimulates it into mounting a response. Vaccines contain antigens.

Attenuated Weakened, but still alive. Attenuated vaccines (sometimes called live attenuated) stimulate an immune response, but without causing the illness.

Autoimmunity A condition where your body's immune system turns on itself, causing disease. A whole galaxy of diseases is now known to be due to autoimmunity, including multiple sclerosis, rheumatoid arthritis, type 1 diabetes, coeliac disease and lupus.

Bacterium A single-celled microorganism, capable of dividing rapidly and causing disease. Whooping cough, tuberculosis, tetanus and diphtheria are all examples of bacterial infections. Bacteriology is the science of studying bacteria.

Cold chain The supply chain that ensures vaccines are kept at a consistent temperature during transport from the factory to the place where they will eventually be given. Most vaccines need to be kept between two and eight degrees centigrade, although some need to be transported frozen.

Conjugate A type of vaccine where the active ingredient, the antigen, is attached to another component, usually a protein, to make it more effective. Some of the meningitis vaccines are conjugates.

Endemic Adjective that describes a disease that occurs all year round, at an expected, predictable rate. For example, malaria is endemic in East Africa.

Epidemic Rapid spread of a disease to a large number of people. A somewhat subjective term, as there isn't a single defined threshold at which a disease becomes an epidemic.

Epidemiology The study of the incidence and distribution diseases, and their causes.

Efficacy A term widely used in medicine, to describe the capacity of a drug or vaccine to achieve a desired effect. The efficacy of a vaccine is the percentage reduction in disease in a vaccinated group of people compared to an unvaccinated group, measured in a clinical trial.

Genome The entire genetic information about an organism.

Herd immunity Indirect protection against an infectious disease, which happens when a high percentage of a population becomes immune, either through having caught the disease or having been vaccinated. Non-immune people are protected because the disease no longer has the ability to spread.

Immune Possessing immunity against an infectious disease, i.e., protected.

Immune system The collective name for all the parts of your body involved in mounting an immune response. The innate immune system is what you are born with, the adaptive immune system is the one that your body learns as you get exposed to different infectious diseases.

Immunisation The act of making someone immune to an infectious disease. The word is often used to describe a vaccine, or the act of being vaccinated, but catching the disease is also a type of immunisation.

Immunogenicity The ability of a vaccine to stimulate an immune response. The more immunogenic the vaccine, the better the immune response.

Immunology The study of the immune system

Inactivated vaccine A vaccine that contains a virus or bacterium that has been killed, so it cannot multiply. Sometimes called a non-replicating vaccine.

Incubation period The length of time between being exposed to an infectious disease and developing symptoms. Usually a few days but can be longer.

Inoculation A rather old-fashioned word which is sometimes used instead of vaccination. It also has a broader meaning of deliberately injecting infectious material, for example you make blue cheese by inoculating it with mould.

Intramuscular The technique of injecting a vaccine into a muscle. This is the most effective method for most vaccines.

Intranasal The technique of squirting a vaccine up the nose.

Latency The ability of a virus or bacteria to remain dormant in the body, only to reactivate later and cause disease. Chickenpox is a good example, appearing later in life as shingles.

Leucocyte The generic term for white blood cells, which are the ones involved in immunity. There are many different types of leucocyte.

Live vaccine A vaccine made from a virus or bacterium that has been weakened, but not killed. They continue to replicate in the body after the vaccine is given. Sometimes called a replicating vaccine.

Lymphocyte A type of white blood cell that specialises in providing immunity to a specific virus or bacterium. There are various types of lymphocytes involved in providing immunity, the most important are called T cells and B cells.

Microbiome The collective term for all the microorganisms, including bacteria, viruses and fungi, which inhabit the body.

Microorganism A living cell, or groups of cells only visible under a microscope. Sometimes called a microbe. Includes viruses, bacteria, protozoa, some fungi and algae.

Oral The technique of giving a vaccine by mouth, i.e., swallowed.

Organism Any living being, including bacteria, viruses, plants and animals.

Pandemic An epidemic that occurs all over the world at the same time. The classical pandemic diseases are plague, cholera and flu. Newer members of the club are HIV and of course COVID-19.

Pathogen A microorganism that can cause an infectious disease. Bacteria, viruses, fungi and protozoa are all examples of pathogens. Pathogenicity is used to describe the disease-causing potential of a microorganism.

Phases 1, 2, 3, 4 The different stages of clinical trials, in the order they are done. The trials get progressively bigger, with more volunteers, at each stage.

Polysaccharide The coat that covers some bacteria, composed of components that are similar to sugar. Some vaccines for meningitis are made with polysaccharides.

Reactogenicity The ability of a vaccine to cause side effects. The more reactogenic, the more side effects the vaccine causes.

Toxin A poison produced by a bacterium that causes symptoms. Diphtheria and tetanus are both toxin-mediated diseases.

Toxoid A type of vaccine, made by killing the toxin of a bacterium.

Vaccination The act of giving someone a vaccine. Often used interchangeably with the word immunisation, which strictly means making someone immune (see above).

Vaccinology The science of the study of vaccines and vaccination. It covers all aspects, including research, manufacturing, and the role of vaccines in society.

Variants Different versions of a virus, which arise by changes in the genetic sequence in the virus. A change in the genetic sequence of the virus is called a mutation, and a variant may contain one or more mutations.

Variolation Early term used to describe the act of deliberately infecting someone with smallpox in order to make them immune.

Vector A vector is another name for a carrier, and is used widely in medicine and science. Some infectious diseases rely on vectors to be transmitted, for example mosquitos are the vector for malaria. There are certain types of vaccines in which a harmless virus is used as a vector to carry genetic material into your body.

Virulence A word used to describe the extent to which a virus or bacterium can cause serious disease.

Virus A tiny microorganism, which causes disease by invading and multiplying in cells. Measles, mumps, rubella, influenza and of course COVID-19 are all examples of viral infections. Virology is the science of studying viruses.

Abbreviations

Ab	Antibody
AE	Adverse event
Ag	Antigen
BCG	Bacille Calmette-Guérin, the vaccine for tuberculosis
CDC	Centers for Disease Control and Prevention. The US agency that monitors infectious diseases and provides guidance on their control
CEPI	Coalition for Epidemic Preparedness Innovations
COVAX	COVID-19 Vaccines Global Access. The organisation, coordinated by the World Health Organization, that was set up to ensure equal access to COVID-19 vaccines around the world
COVID-19	COronavirus VIrus Disease, 2019
DNA	Deoxyribonucleic acid. The genetic material that stores all the information about you
DPT	Diphtheria/Pertussis/Tetanus
EMA	European Medicines Agency, the EU agency that licenses and regulates drugs, devices and vaccines
FDA	Food and Drug Administration, the equivalent US agency

Gavi   The Vaccine Alliance (previously the Global Alliance for Vaccines and Immunization). Partnership between the World Health Organization, UNICEF, the World Bank, and the Bill and Melinda Gates Foundation that aims to increase access to vaccines in poor countries

HAV   Hepatitis A virus

HBV   Hepatitis B virus

HPV   Human Papillomavirus , the virus that causes cancer of the cervix

Hib   *Haemophilus influenzae* type b, a bacterium that causes a type of meningitis

IDMC   Independent Data Monitoring Committee, the team that independently checks a large clinical trial, particularly to look for side effects. Sometimes called a Data and Safety Monitoring Board (DSMB)

IPV   Inactivated polio vaccine

MHRA   Medicines and Healthcare products Regulatory Agency. The UK agency that licenses and regulates drugs, devices and vaccines

MMR   Measles/Mumps/Rubella

OPV   Oral polio vaccine

RNA   Ribonucleic acid. The genetic material that converts the information stored in your DNA, in order to make proteins

R_0 The basic reproduction number, often called simply the R number, which is the measure of how easily an infectious disease can be transmitted to others

SAE   Serious adverse event

UNICEF   United Nations Children's Fund. The agency that provides developmental and humanitarian aid to children, worldwide

WHO   World Health Organization

Index

Printed in the United States
by Baker & Taylor Publisher Services